# Stem Cells for Spinal Stenosis



ISBN: 978-1-963592-10-8
ISBN: 978-1-963592-11-5
ISBN: 978-1-963592-12-2

Published by Will Bozeman



For more information:

**http://www.willbozeman.com**

# Table of Contents

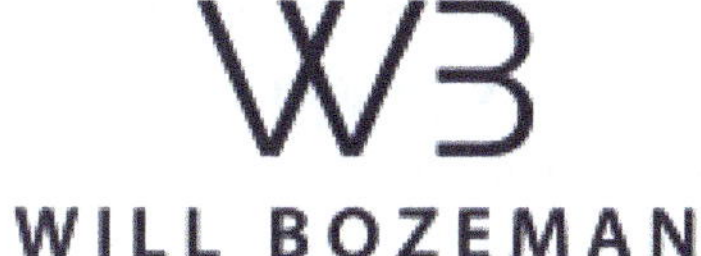

 Willbozeman.com

 Will@willbozeman.com

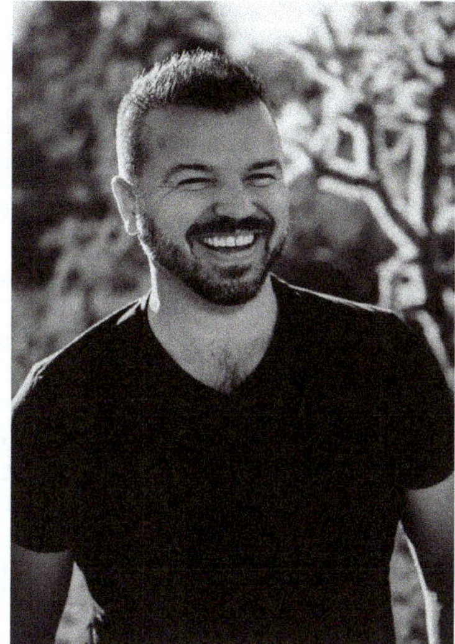

Will is a healthcare executive, innovator, entrepreneur, inventor, and writer with a wide range of experience in the medical field. Will has multiple degrees in a wide range of subjects that give depth to his capability as an entrepreneur and capacity to operate as an innovative healthcare executive. Will has an associate degree in electrical technology, two undergraduate degrees in biotechnology and archaeology, an MBA, and attended medical school in Alabama.

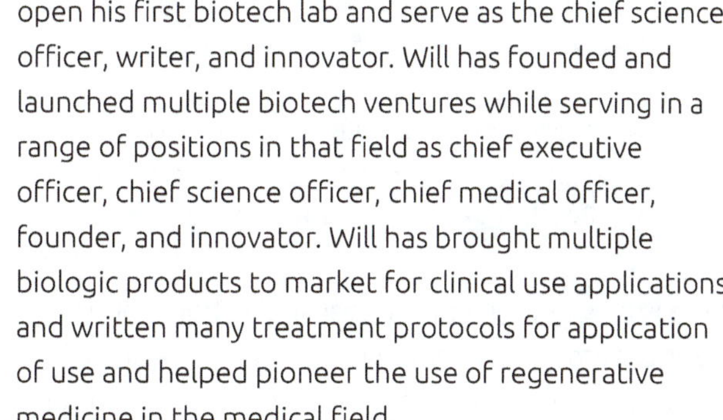

Will took a leave of absence from medical school to open his first biotech lab and serve as the chief science officer, writer, and innovator. Will has founded and launched multiple biotech ventures while serving in a range of positions in that field as chief executive officer, chief science officer, chief medical officer, founder, and innovator. Will has brought multiple biologic products to market for clinical use applications and written many treatment protocols for application of use and helped pioneer the use of regenerative medicine in the medical field.

**If you've already read one of my stem cell books, you'll notice the first two chapters are the same. Just skip to chapter 3 if you want to jump straight into the main topic! Though, a refresher on the first two chapters never hurt anyone either.**

# Prologue

What an exciting age of medicine we live in today!

Stem cells and stem cell applications are already one of the greatest discoveries of modern medicine, and the vast majority of our advanced stem cell medical applications and uses are yet to come.

At the time of writing, there are countless studies on the clinical and medical application of stem cells from very specific disease conditions like specific cancers and congenital diseases, to more general use stem cell treatments for systemic inflammation, anti-aging and longevity, and even for use in aesthetic treatments like high-end facials, skin rejuvenation, and hair regrowth.

Of course, some of the really interesting applications that researchers have their eyes on these days are advancements in nerve tissue regeneration and organ tissue growth and development.

I, for one, am excited for the day when we can simply grow organs for replacement instead of having a transplant list. Also, how about treating a range of chronic illnesses with a simple IV stem cell application on a regular basis?

There is no shortage of potential applications for use. However, for the purposes of this book, I want to zero in on what is happening and available right now, what is available to patients in the United States, and what is available at the international stem cell treatment level.

**My background and history in regenerative medicine**

My background in stem cell biotechnology began with my biotech undergraduate degree, where I performed a range of cellular biotech functions, culturing and expanding various cell lines and isolating cellular DNA, and I conducted a range of lab testing procedures to prepare us for the exciting world of cellular biotech.

One of my favorite undergraduate projects that really helped me understand the details of the science of cellular biotechnology was to build a new cell culture lab for our university biotech department.

This project really opened my eyes to how a cell culture lab worked and operated from start to finish. I didn't just learn how to do only specific tasks, like most students; I learned how everything worked, and the how and why behind it.

I learned all about the current state of the industry because I had to build the lab. I had to order and test equipment; determine capabilities and functional uses; troubleshoot lab problems, operations and activity flow of the lab; determine the capabilities of what could be produced in a cell culture lab; and, of course, understand where the industry needed innovation and what was on the horizon.

Most students only got a tiny window into this world, but I was able to stand in front of a huge bay window and see what cellular biotech was all about. This is what really helped me understand the foundation of the world of regenerative medicine and started me down the path of stem cell therapy and regenerative medical applications.

Biotechnology is a notoriously risky field to be in because the people who are often exceptional with the science are not often exceptional with the business and practical applications. Luckily, I snagged my MBA before medical school, so I have a little more understanding of the business of a biotech operation and how to make it succeed.

It doesn't matter how lofty or noble your biotech ambitions are, if you can't pay your bills, you can't do anything to further your efforts … and people don't seem to like working for free.

Business and biotech are highly intertwined. Because there are so many variables to account for, biotechnology remains one of the more difficult categories of business to engage in, and yet it continues to attract hundreds and even thousands of new startups and ventures every year.

I believe this is because of the allure of the magnitude of what can be accomplished or what could be developed if your idea succeeds.

The potential upside for success is more enticing than the risk/fear of failure. I've felt this strange dynamic many times. I'm looking at a potentially life-saving therapy and I can immediately convince myself that I would sacrifice my own financial security to get this treatment to market!

I tell you this because this new era of amazing medical therapy is brought to you by innovators and pioneers in this field who often ride the edge of success all the way to the end, good or bad.

Particularly in the world of stem cells, the people I meet are not just thinking of how to start a business or get a good job, they are thinking of how to change the world. The potential for stem cell therapy to revolutionize many categories of medicine is very strong, and this is what drives everyone in this field.

I myself am guilty of diving headfirst into biotech startups because the potential benefits and applications are so exciting that I can't say no. To the surprise of my professors, I started my first lab company, stem cell processing, and storage lab while I was in my biotech undergrad program.

It provided private processing and cryopreservation storage of cord blood and tissue for later stem cell therapies for parents who wanted that protection and assurance for their children. My professors hadn't seen many students apply what they had learned so quickly in real life. I found myself in real-world conversations with professors over my company and the potential growth and expansion of my startup.

I had conversations with my professors, literally on the side of the classroom, discussing investment and growth options while other students completed their regular course work. I tell you this because my undergrad experience was completely different from that of my peers.

This particular lab operation to process and store cord blood stem cells for parents having children who wanted to save those cells was more than just a business venture; I saw it as a calling, my first real life stem cell operation.

Cord blood stem cells provide a specific type of stem cell that could become valuable to a patient if they develop certain medical conditions down the road, but the only sure fire way to know you have a match available when you need it is to bank it yourself for later.

When I started this company, it was still very new in the market and the pushback was actually from the doctors in the hospital who didn't want to be bothered with having to collect the cord blood.

Even though they usually aren't the ones doing it – it's almost always a nurse or medical assistant doing the actual collection – they still didn't like that it was a "new thing" to have to deal with.

I'll never forget the comment from the doctor who delivered our first child, regarding our collection of cord blood. "If we have time, we'll try to get to your science experiment." He referred to it as a frivolous science experiment and was annoyed that he had to be bothered with it. He was an older doctor and likely was not ready for this new world of advanced stem cell therapy.

A few years later I spoke to the partner in that same obstetrics office, and he said they had seen multiple children whose lives had been saved by cord blood banking and he was now an advocate for cord blood storage.

His partner had mocked it only a few years before that, then suddenly it hit them that it's not just a science experiment, but an advanced lifesaving medical protocol. Suddenly, the world they worked in was new and different, and people who previously would not have been alive were now alive because of it. It happened that fast.

I continued that lab venture into medical school but had to hand it off to a colleague due to time constraints: med school is pretty busy. I was halfway through medical school when I was invited to co-venture and open a biotech lab focusing on stem cell processing and stem cell product manufacture for medical use by physicians in the orthopedic and pain management space.

I took a leave of absence from medical school to be the chief science and medical officer for this biotech venture and opened this new biotech lab in Arizona, one of the hubs of biotech in the nation at that time.

I was already through the academics of medical school, and I realized two things pretty quickly. Firstly, what I was being taught was so far behind what I had already studied in biotech that if I wanted to be at the forefront of medical innovation, I would not get there by traditional medical school processes for at least a decade.

Secondly, I could do so much more good in the medical world through my experience in biotechnology and business experience than I would finishing medical school and going into residency for several more years.

I saw the writing on the wall pretty quickly and chose the path of biotech and innovation. I'll forever be grateful for the medical knowledge I gained from my academic years in medical school; this education has greatly helped me in the process.

I'll always advocate for education, but there's a point where you know what you know, you know what other people don't know, you know what you can do and what other people can't do or aren't doing, and you start seeing the opportunities where you can make a larger impact.

It took several months of contemplation to not go back and finish med school, but my path was already being structured for me through successful efforts in this new biotech venture I'd left med school for. I never looked back, and I have directly seen my positive impact at the national level in the field of regenerative medicine.

I built a tissue processing lab in Arizona and developed multiple product lines and lectured on stem cells and clinical applications at multiple medical conferences before my med school colleagues were finished with school.

As of the time of writing, I have started multiple biotech companies, multiple medical companies, built/owned/operated multiple clinical labs, developed dozens of products and services in the medical field, and written hundreds of pages of scientifically backed content for these operations and for product use in the medical field.

I have also written numerous treatment protocols for the application of regenerative medicine products in medical practice, and I've personally taught and coached hundreds of physicians and medical providers on the use and application of biologic products and many other aspects of the field of regenerative medicine, resulting in the direct application of therapy to tens of thousands of patients.

I would say that one of my greater achievements in this space has been the education, coaching, and awareness I've brought to hundreds of physicians around the nation. This has probably done more to advance regenerative medicine than anything else I could have done during those years after I left medical school.

I'm excited to bring this guidebook to you for your personal education on your options for the various regenerative medicine treatments available in the United States and in the international medical field.

Let's dive in!

# Chapter 1 - Stem Cells

## Stem Cells 101

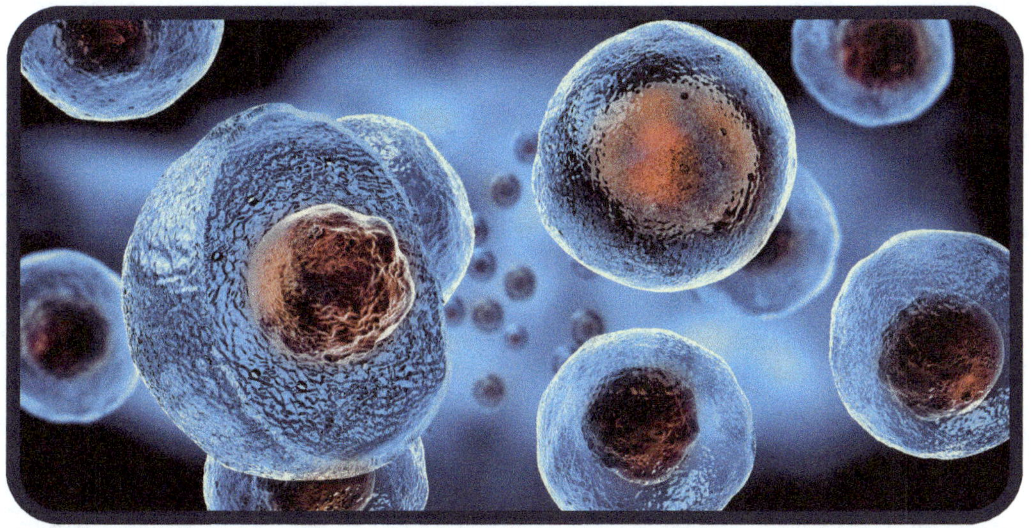

A stem cell is the foundation unit of cellular growth and development. It's basically a blank slate cell that can grow in any direction it needs for cellular development of the whole body.

The remarkable behavior of a stem cell is that when it divides into two cells, one cell will divert off into the type of cell it needs to become, and the remaining cell stays a stem cell and can split again and again to produce more and more cells as needed.

This process of a stem cell splitting into a new specialized type of cell is called differentiation - the process of becoming different. It's a nice scientific word for a stem cell changing into a different cell type, and you'll hear it a lot because it's the fundamental aspect of what makes stem cells so amazing; the secret sauce of why stem cells are so useful.

Stem cells differentiate over and over and over. This is where it really gets interesting. How long can this go on? How long can stem cells keep dividing and creating a new dedicated cell line while the original one stays a stem cell? Turns out, basically your whole life, though it slows down and there are DNA mechanisms for how long it can do this.

Telomeres are the ends of a DNA strand and are the most commonly discussed aspect of cellular replication because telomere length can determine how many times a cell can replicate.

Telomeres don't code for things, but they make it possible for the rest of the DNA to work. This replication declining mechanism has been identified as, and believed to be, a source and ultimate cause of aging and age-related illnesses.

Simply put, telomeres measure our life span and capacity to age and die. As just mentioned, a telomere is the extra end string of DNA left over after a cell has replicated its DNA. The easiest way to describe a telomere is this: you tie a shoestring, but you don't tie the knot at the very end, you tie it down where the strings meet the braid.

You then have nice long strings left over. You need that long string in order to tie another knot, because you can't tie a good knot using a short string. Also, you still need a nice tight knot with no dangling strands, so you cut off the extra length of string hanging off that knot. That's how telomeres get shorter with each replication cycle.

Over time, each replication shaves a little DNA off the end of that string, so eventually there's no telomere string left to tie knots with. But you still need to tie those knots, so you start tying knots with actual DNA that codes for important things.

That DNA is now being chopped off the ends as well, just like telomeres were before, and you start losing valuable DNA. This is the beginning of the end of that DNA strand. After a while, that shoe is barely hanging on and will most likely fall off with a little too much activity.

This simplified description helps explain how telomeres are associated with stem cell activity. The question of how long a stem cell can replicate is a bit more complex, but it's really easy to understand that there is a limit. Now you know two terms: differentiation and telomeres. You're on your way to being a stem cell expert!

The entire story of stem cells is a little more than I want to get into in this book, but what I do want to discuss is the category of stem cells that is currently applicable to medical use. These two basic concepts of differentiation and telomeres really summarize why we need stem cells in medicine.

After a while, you just aren't going to make enough cells fast enough to replace the aging/dying/damaged cells in your body, and that is why everyone should be extremely excited about the new field of stem cell medicine.

You obviously want to learn about the tremendous advantages stem cell therapies have for average medical conditions. After all, this is a guidebook to stem cell therapy for a specific medical condition you're interested in learning about, so it makes sense that I get to brass tacks on this.

# Stem Cell Types

**Hematopoietic stem cells:** (he-mat-o-poi-et-ic) Hematopoietic stem cells differentiate into blood-based cells. Heme is the medical scientific word for iron, and the medical word for anything to do with blood, because iron makes your blood red and transports oxygen.

For example, hematology is the study of blood, so that should help you remember that hematopoietic stem cells make your blood cells. Most stem cell therapies you'll hear about in the coming years are NOT hematopoietic based therapies, and that's why I wanted to mention them first and then put them aside while I get to the more popular and more diverse category of mesenchymal stem cells.

**Mesenchymal stem cells:** (mess-en-ky-mal) Mesenchymal stem cells differentiate into many other cell types. One of these types is musculoskeletal tissue, also known medically as MSK.

MSK tissue contains cells such as cartilage, bone, muscle, tendons, and connective tissues, which are of particular interest in regenerative medicine because there are so many conditions in this category that can be treated.

You need to remember the initialism MSK because this is what is used most of the time to describe this category. This means mesenchymal stem cells are the type that can regenerate tissues for all the various injuries we endure through the daily activities of life.

Everything from spinal stenosis and osteoarthritis to serious spinal injuries would look to mesenchymal stem cells as a possible treatment.

In order to explain the treatment possibilities with mesenchymal stem cells, there are two more terms I want to teach you here: autologous and allogeneic. Autologous means it comes from you; allogeneic means it comes from someone else and is given to you. These two terms define the entire state of stem cell therapy in the US and internationally.

See, you are really becoming a stem cell expert because most people have no idea those two terms exist or what they mean, much less that those two terms are how the world of stem cell therapy is divided up.

**What is and what is not an actual stem cell treatment?**

Buckle in and I'll run through a snap account of the regenerative medicine product portfolio in the market today. I'll follow up after this on where you're likely to see and hear about these different products and therapies, what to look for, and what to avoid.

# Stem Cell Treatments and Products

The first thing you have to know is that the term "stem cells" became a common vernacular term for any regenerative product because it was the preferred term to use. This is because it was such a high-end medical term and because there were so many different products, it was hard to explain the differences, so everyone just called everything stem cells.

This caused a lot of confusion and, ultimately, got the attention of the FDA and the FTC; I'll explain those details later.

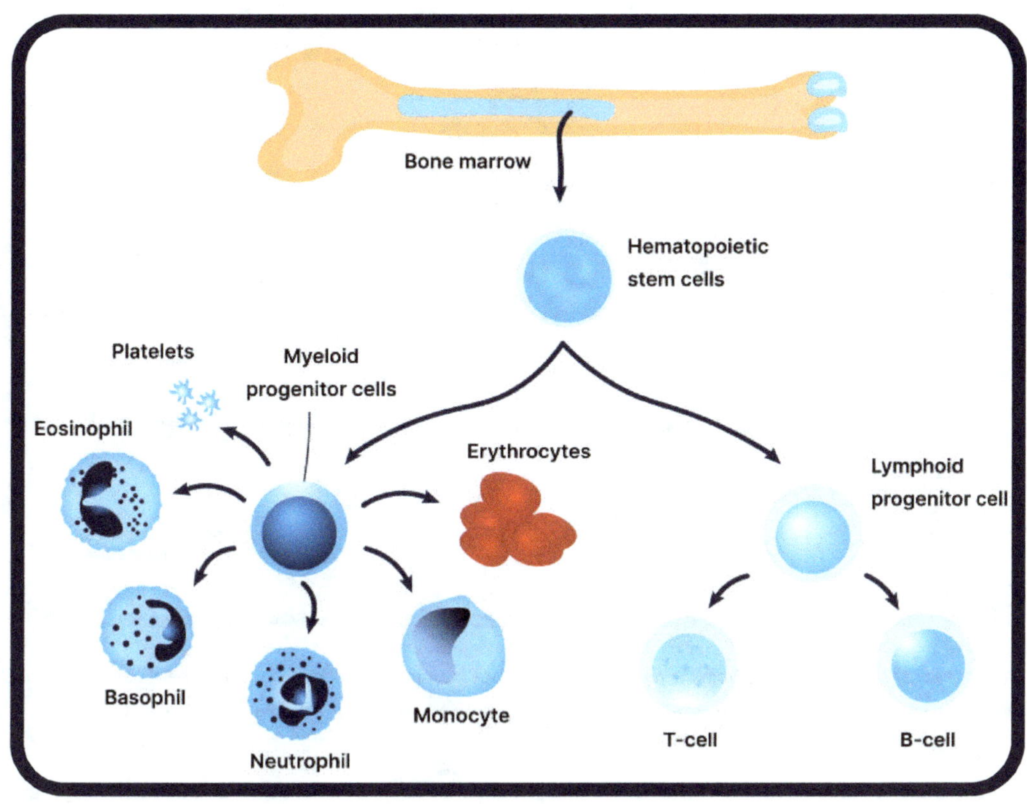


*Hematopoietic stem cells, derived from the bone marrow, proliferating and differentiating into any type of blood cell.*

*Data from:* https://researchfeatures.com/steady-state-hematopoietic-stem-cells-transplantation/

**Bone marrow stem cells:** (autologous) Bone marrow stem cells are collected from your own bone marrow, processed, refined and concentrated, and reinjected into the target treatment areas. This is considered the traditional standard stem cell treatment in the US, and this was the gold standard for treating musculoskeletal conditions for the last couple of decades.

The downsides are that it requires a moderately uncomfortable procedure to collect bone marrow aspirate stem cells (BMAC), and the cells are technically as old as you are, so that whole section on telomeres now starts to make sense; your own stem cells are not any younger than you are.

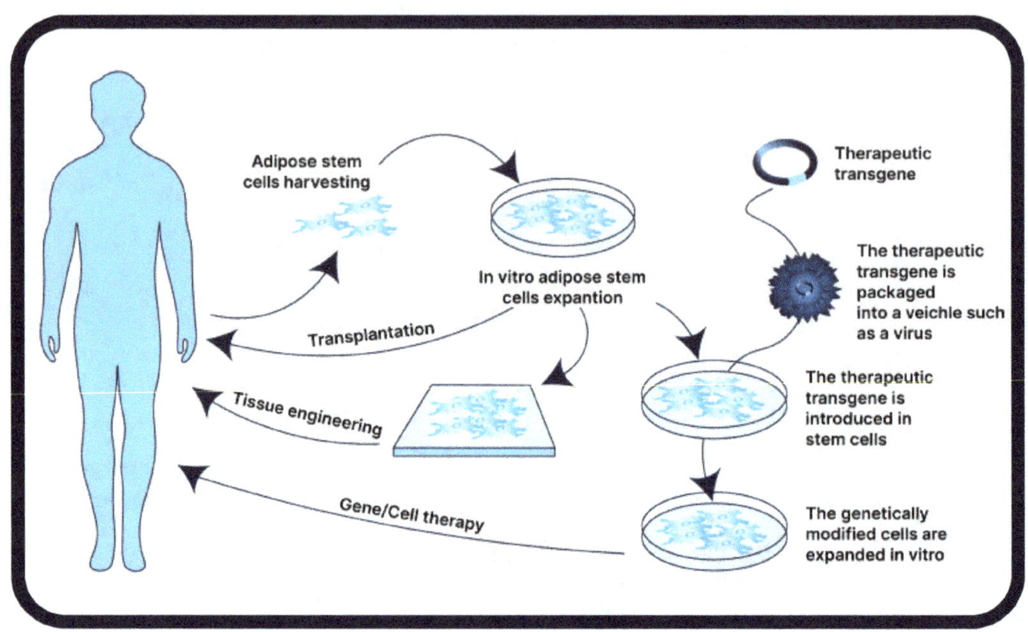


*Hematopoietic stem cells, derived from the bone marrow, proliferating and differentiating into any type of blood cell.*
*Data from: https://researchfeatures.com/steady-state-hematopoietic-stem-cells-transplantation/*

Adipose stem cells: Adipose stem cells are stem cells collected from your fat tissue through a liposuction procedure. These are becoming more popular for several reasons, but ultimately, it has been a battleground for regenerative medicine advocates because of legal issues and unscrupulous medical offices making claims of a wide range of cures.

I am no expert on the latest in this legal and compliance battle but I read about it and hear about it often.

Remember, even a product that works can fail if the people using it make unsubstantiated claims, are abusive in their marketing tactics, or are abusive in pricing the treatment. Also, this requires liposuction to collect the fat and harvest the cells, so it's still invasive.

Ultimately, it needs to be an available tool in the stem cell treatment category, so I'm hoping it continues its path to better compliance and standardization.

**Cultured expanded stem cells:** This is my favorite category of stem cell treatment because it's THE future of stem cell therapy worldwide.

Cultured and expanded stem cells are grown in specialized cell culture labs and can be grown using autologous or allogeneic stem cells. So you can use your bone marrow stem cells and grow them out to get a proper high dose for treatment, or you can use compliant perinatal tissue stem cells. You can isolate and grow a tremendous quantity of specific mesenchymal stem cells and have enough for multiple treatments all at the same time.

The ultimate problem with bone marrow or adipose cells is that you can only get so much material, so you can only create enough high dose stem cell content for limited use. Cell expansion is the future of stem cell treatment because you can grow just about as much as you need or want.

Also, with advanced techniques, you can stimulate stem cells to differentiate into other cell types in the culture process.

Think: growing a batch of cardiac stem cells specifically for heart repair, or a batch of cartilage tissue stem cells for joint injuries! Also, think: lab grown organs and tissues. This is THE advantage in stem cell medicine and therapy and the future of cellular medicine as it becomes more formalized and standardized for predictable outcomes.

This is much more efficient than personal autologous collection methods like bone marrow or adipose collection procedures. The reason we see so much bone marrow and adipose activity in the US is because cultured expanded cells are prohibited in the US medical system.

This is mostly for good reasons though, as it's very complicated to get it right and it needs to be refined and standardized for wide-scale application.

Standardizing cellular therapy is not like other manufactured medications or treatments where chemistry can replicate the same molecule perfectly. Cell culture is like trying to encourage the cells to replicate the way you want, but you can't always count on it to be a perfect replication process.

This is why it's hard to regulate cultured cell therapies, but the industry is getting much better at these processes.

I intend to be a part of the cellular therapy standardization process in the US because it's definitely the future of medicine, but I don't want it to be in a field that is bombarded with bad actors trying to game the market.

As of this writing, I am working with my team on some of these standardized cultured expanded stem cell therapies with plans and hopes to conduct trials and help get these treatments through the approval process in the US.

As luck would have it, several groups are already experts in cultured expanded cell therapies on the international level, so you can still get these procedures done today – just outside the US – and the applications are amazing! The range of conditions being treated with startling outcomes is very exciting.

At any time while reading this book, you can reach out to me and I'll direct you to some of the best options for this around the world.

Obviously, the MSK category is already a highly popular category, but now we are seeing movement into treatments for things like COPD (chronic obstructive pulmonary disease), heart tissue repair, neural tissue repair, eye and ocular healing and repair, advanced esthetics and hair regeneration, and, of course, one of my favorites, longevity and anti-aging therapies through full-body inflammation reduction via IV stem cell therapy.

There are a lot of other really exciting things, but I don't want to suggest that these conditions are being cured with these stem cell treatments yet. Some treatment types are helping these people and, in many cases, it's about the only available option that will work, even if it's a modest result.

I personally knew a retired medical doctor who sought treatment for his chronic condition. I don't want to say what it was because I don't want to suggest that what he did will work for anyone else, nor that cultured expanded cell therapy will treat or cure this particular condition or act as a treatment option just yet, but he had very impressive results and I almost didn't believe it.

Unfortunately, this treatment only curbed the symptoms, which is still amazing for what it was able to do for him. The condition came back eventually, but the severity of his symptoms was significantly reduced and mostly resolved for nearly a year after that treatment.

I can think of many people and many conditions where if there was a routine annual stem cell treatment that only reduced the severity of the symptoms, it would still be a tremendous success and would become the new standard of care for that condition.

His results were something I didn't believe would happen at all. I knew the guy decently well; he was a retired family practice doctor. So our conversations on his treatment process were very interesting. He made me believe that what they are saying they're able to do in the international stem cell treatment market is actually possible using cultured expanded stem cell therapies.

I know it's exciting, but it's still a very new field so I'm not suggesting or claiming that any condition I mention or discuss is curable or can be cured with these treatments ... yet. I simply believe it is the right track to a better future of medical treatment.

**Birth tissue stem cell products:** Immediately, I want to point out that the birth tissue stem cell products I'm talking about here come from perfectly ethical and legally donated tissues that come from normal, healthy Cesarean section deliveries by donors who are fully informed about the procedure and go through rigorous and regulated vetting, screening, and testing.

I know a lot about this process as I've launched multiple companies and labs that made these birth-tissue-based regenerative products. The best way to think of how this is compliant and moral and ethical is to understand that during a regular C-section delivery, the mother and the baby are safe and healthy and they both move on with their lives as normal, but what about all the leftover birth tissues involved in the process?

Those tissues are normally disposed of as medical waste, but they are perfectly healthy tissues that can be repurposed into something useful. This is exactly what the perinatal birth tissue category has accomplished, using healthy, safe tissues that are safely, ethically, and morally collected and processed into useful medical products. It's a wonderful way to make something useful out of something that would otherwise be useless.

All the collection programs I worked with in my career were heavily regulated by the FDA and a very detailed paper trail was in place for each tissue collection we received. I've explained the appropriateness of this category of tissue collection to hundreds of doctors and patients.

Everyone is skeptical after hearing about some of the bad actors in the industry mentioned in news articles. I'd be skeptical, too, if I hadn't actually been in the middle of this process for so long. I've seen so much good come from this treatment category, and, of course, where there's good there's going to be a few bad actors exploiting that good.

There is a range of products created from perinatal birth tissues. Two of the primary reasons birth tissues are so useful are: first, the cells are brand new, so they are young and active and have a full life cycle of replication potential, if you recall the topic of telomeres and stem cell replication lifespan.

The second reason is that the cells in the tissues have little to no detectable immunomarkers on the cells. This means that you don't have to type match a donor to a recipient like you do with blood and organs. I've explained this concept to several hundred doctors over my biotech career because, to the average trained physician, our cells have markers that identify ourselves versus foreign cells.

The short answer to why these tissues have little to no detectable immunomarkers is that the mother and the developing baby are two unique entities with their own identifying immunity markers. So if they could sense each other's presence, they'd fight each other with their own immune responses.

Birth tissues like the placenta, umbilical cord, and amniotic membrane are created specifically to overcome this problem by being immune marker neutral tissues. The amniotic fluid, membrane, umbilical cord, and placenta are designed to shield the two entities from each other, thus making the tissues ideal for use as stem cell sources because the cells won't have immune markers to trigger responses.

**Here's a list of the different birth tissues that are popular for stem cell collection:**

Industry note: *At the time of writing, all birth tissue injectable biologics are being reclassified under FDA regulations, so you may not see many of these in the market anymore until regulators iron out how they will be allowed moving forward.*

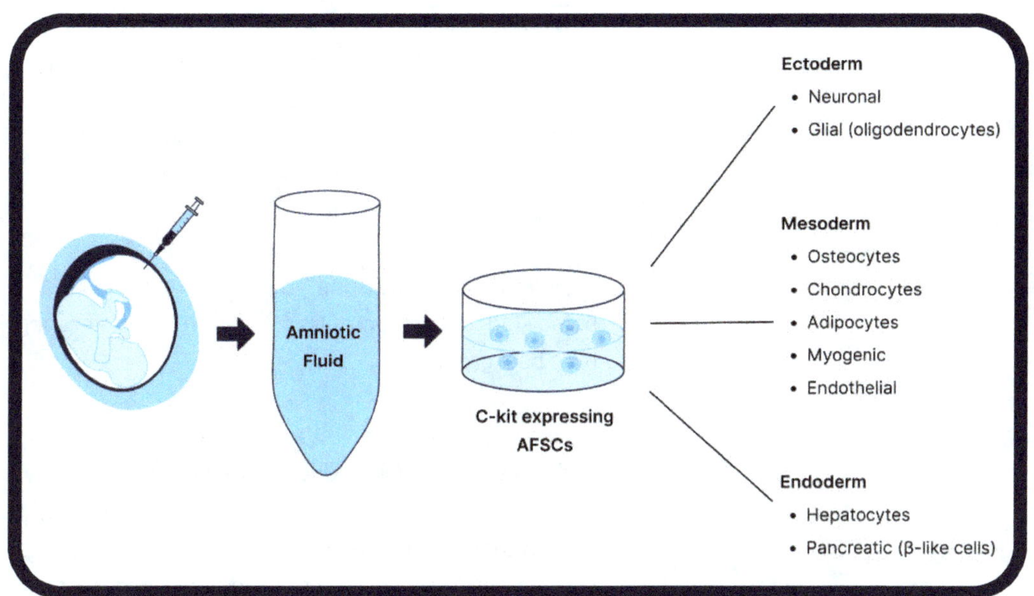


*Amniotic fluid stem cell isolation and differentiation.*

*Data from: https://www.researchgate.net/figure/Amniotic-fluid-stem-cell-AFSC-isolation-and-differentiation-Cells-are-collected-via_fig1_342967332*

Amniotic fluid stem cells: This is the actual fluid that the fetus floated in and lived in during development. Naysayers love to claim this is just baby urine, but I've only ever heard this argument when a doctor is trying to sell you what they're offering, that isn't amniotic fluid.

Also, with all the studies on amniotic fluid in recent years, they've been proven wildly incorrect over the last decade for trying to suggest that amniotic fluid is mere baby urine. Again, they're only saying that if they're trying to sell you something else.

Whether intentionally selling something else or unintentionally due to lack of education on the details, it's not the same world we lived in 20 years ago when it comes to understanding biologics.

Though it's true that babies do "urinate" a mild diluted version of urine in amniotic fluid, they also continuously drink amniotic fluid as well because it is completely safe for the fetus to consume, and this fluid is filled with high levels of a wide range of growth factors and nutrients. It's nature's perfect regenerative fluid.

Remember that the baby's actual harmful waste is removed through the mother via the umbilical cord, not via the baby, so all the harmful elements of urine waste have to be removed so they do not concentrate in the baby's liquid waste where it would build up to dangerous levels in amniotic fluid.

So, if you hear "baby urine," then you know you're being sold, or the doctor isn't very solid on their regen med background.

However, I like to look at it as an opportunity to learn and grow. After all, I taught hundreds of doctors a wide range of regen med topics over the years that helped them apply therapies to patients. They have to start somewhere, and most of the time the doctors I taught were starting from scratch. I applaud them for leaping into the future!

**Will's Industry Insight #1:**
*Ultimately, after 30,000+ cases using products created in my labs throughout my biotech career, the general consensus from the doctors and practices I've worked with is that fresh frozen amniotic fluid works better and produces better and longer outcomes.*

Amniotic fluid comes in two main forms: fresh frozen and room temperature sterilized. I've worked with many versions of both and seen amazing outcomes with both for many years.

There may be a few viable stem cells in fresh amniotic fluid by the time it's injected into a patient, but nowhere near enough to justify calling it a stem cell injection, not to mention that many amniotic fluid products intentionally screen out the cell content.

**Will's Industry Insight #2:**
*Genuine amniotic fluid is not considered a stem cell product, yet it has been routinely called stem cells as a commonly used vernacular term by doctors and pretty much everyone else in the industry. Now you can see how easy it is to confuse the different names of treatments and confuse patients on what they're getting.*

Also, when a doctor or medical office says their product has millions of stem cells, and they're located in the US, they're talking about general cell content, NOT stem cell counts.

What percentage of cells in these tissues are actual stem cells? It varies, but in amniotic fluid, for example, about 2-3% of the cell content is actual stem cells; the rest are all sorts of other tissue cells.

In the US, we are not allowed to refine and concentrate stem cells out of birth tissues into a concentrated injection, so if the doctor is taking a vial out of the freezer, you're not getting a vial full of stem cells, you're getting a vial full of a homogenous tissue composed of mostly non-stem cells and tissue particulates, an injection with very few stem cells that most likely will not be viable living healthy cells by the time they are injected.

So, you can see how this is misleading if a medical office is advertising stem cell treatments and claims to have high quantities of stem cells in the injection. That's outright misleading and that's what has gotten the attention of the FDA and gotten the Federal Trade Commission, FTC, involved in regulating what doctors say to patients and what biotech labs and sales reps say to doctors.

**Will's Industry Insight #3:**
*"Is my doctor selling me a certain number of cells?" If you're in the US then the short answer is no, not really, at least not really stem cells. Again, being a biotech founder, product developer, and manufacturer, and working closely with hundreds of doctors gives you a lot of insight into how easy it is to misunderstand what the product is and how to describe it to a patient.*

Despite the lack of genuine stem cell quantities in ready-to-go products in the US market, here's the real kicker you won't hear from your doctor or medical office: pure acellular amniotic fluid works as well as or better than cellular-based injections ... without any cell content!

You won't hear that from the office trying to sell you a treatment based on stem cell counts or stem cell viability content, but I've seen and heard this many times in offices that do a lot of treatment volume. This is what actually led me to create an acellular product line in the first place - to make a pure amniotic fluid product with no cell content. It worked tremendously well and outperformed a wide range of other products that claimed to have cell content.

As I mentioned before, if it's in the US and they're advertising an allogeneic stem cell product, aka a frozen, ready-to-go injection taken out of the freezer, with a specified cell count, they are not being honest with you about what you're buying, or the doctors themselves are not aware of what they are selling.

Either way, you're not getting what you think you're getting. Aside from that, the assumption for years was that the relatively few viable stem cells in the product were what produced the amazing outcomes everyone was seeing.

Despite the debate over cell content, most doctors I've worked with claim they see as good or better outcomes with pure fluid with no cell content. So, you can see that cells or no cells, it works. So it really does matter what the doctor is selling you and that you're aware of what you're paying for.

But for your own peace of mind, that product you did get injected with will probably work well and these nuances won't really matter. It just helps shape the background of the industry we are in to understand all these details.

**Will's Industry Insight #4:**
*They all work about the same anyway! Most birth tissue products have roughly the same outcomes, despite what tissue they're derived from, or the cell counts, or anything else. I've talked to many doctors about this, and they all agree that the outcome differences between one type and another are nominal, meaning the differences are nominal, but the outcomes are good across the board.*

*So ... why the range of products? The ability to make a different product and stand out in the biotech market is a possibility for any biotech company, so it's attractive to create a unique product rather than just copy another. This was a very common practice for years and created the "Wild West" of new biologic regenerative medicine products.*

**Will's Industry Insight #5:**
*Everything your doctor knows about stem cells, they've learned from a sales rep, or at least this was the norm for years and years. It's an unfortunate truth that the vast majority of what you're hearing in the doctor's office was taught by a sales rep for whatever product company is selling the product, and it did not come from medical education or personal research by the doctor.*

Unfortunately, it's too easy to just call everything stem cells, but I believe once you attach a price to that stem cell quantity claim you're making, you have to be able to verify that claim, and doctors can't do that in the office, nor can the labs do that once it's in the doctor's office and out of the lab setting. Call it what it is and let the results speak for themselves because the results are still great, they just need to get the messaging right.

I've been asked/recruited/petitioned vigorously by multiple labs and startups to help them create unique birth tissue products to take to market. They all want something they can call their own, something unique, something different, ultimately so they can corner the market on that one type of product that is unique to them.

It's not all bad for companies to want something special. It really is the driver of innovation and positive change in this industry. Because of this drive to innovate novel products, we've landed on some amazing products in the market and the possibility that there will be FDA-approved products in the coming years. It's all spurred by competition and the drive to make something new.

Stem cells are such a new field, doctors don't get educated on it in medical school. I know because I asked about it specifically and my med school professors told me it wasn't a viable subject to teach yet because it was so new.

While they were saying those words in class, I was actively developing the product manufacturing process for my first biotech product venture to isolate cell-rich tissues and make injectable products. We were seeing tremendous results with this product all while my professors wouldn't even acknowledge these as viable treatment options.

So where do the doctors learn about it while in practice? Pretty much from the sales reps making rounds in their offices. Now, I won't go into how risky this is, but I know exactly how these companies craft their products and messages to appear better, unique, different, and something extra special, and, in some cases, something that they actually aren't, as I've stated above.

That said, I can tell in about five seconds if a doctor is reciting sales material education to me or if they know what they are talking about. I had my own set of questions I'd ask that would "prove out" the doctor as reciting sales rep info as their own knowledge.

So I can say from experience that most of the doctors I've talked to, who endeavored to be in the regenerative medicine space, learned everything they know about it from sales reps. Don't even get me started on the sales reps and product distributors in the market.

Most of the reps I've talked to couldn't speak to stem cells or regen med beyond what is printed on the brochure. Some of them are earnest and trying to do good and earn a living, others not so much.

I used to indulge these reps when they wanted to sell me on their company's products or try to recruit me to their company, and I've been the secret shopper for doctors trying to learn the details of a product and been on those phone calls or even in the office to hear the pitch and ask the "hard questions" that the rep should know if they know anything at all.

Some of the doctors I've helped have connected with me for years to help them evaluate a new company or product, needing someone to make sense of the confusion in the market for them.

Additionally, the risky part is that these are usually not professional sales reps like salaried employees who speak for the company, but commission-only sales reps who were never actually medically trained, have never operated professionally in the medical space, or, in some cases, never went to college, and here they are "teaching" doctors about stem cell treatments because they have a brochure.

That's why I push for doctors to do their own research and read their own white papers on the subject.

**Will's Industry Insight #6:**
*"My chiropractor said 'stem cells' were reimbursed by Medicare." How many times have I heard this from patients? I stopped keeping count. Hundreds of doctors and chiropractors around the nation billed insurance and Medicare for "stem cell" products that were never reimbursable in the first place.*

*I've been on dozens of calls to explain why they couldn't do this and what the risk was going to be, and they preferred to believe the commissioned sales rep because what they were saying was more exciting ... and profitable. So, no, currently you can't get your stem cells reimbursed by Medicare, and the doctors and chiropractic offices who are telling patients this are incorrect.*

I could go into the specific details of why this wasn't allowed, but the short answer is that it's pretty clear in the reimbursement system that there is no reimbursement for unapproved biologics, and if you get reimbursement on it, those payers like Medicare and commercial insurers can come and take that money back from the medical office later, after they figure out that the product and treatment weren't covered.

This is not necessarily a problem for patients to deal with, but it can destroy a medical office if they get all that reimbursement clawed back later, which I've seen many times. So it's just a matter of time. I've literally had dozens of calls with offices and billing companies about the risk of them trying to bill for these products.

I actually pleaded with one doctor who was a friend of mine not to do this. He acted like he'd found this secret success in being able to bill insurances for these treatments. He didn't listen to me.

He got clawed back by multiple insurances all at the same time and he had to shut down his office. It was sad, but I tried my best. Fortunately, one of my other friends took my advice and avoided it. Then he called me a few months later to thank me for keeping him out of all that mess.

**Will's Industry Insight #7:**
*"What's the deal with chiropractors selling stem cells?" Yep, I know it doesn't make sense at all, but I can explain. I'll add a disclaimer to this by saying that many chiropractors don't apply to the following category of activity and that I have good friends who are chiropractors who also bemoan the reputation some chiropractors create in the market on this topic.*

Chiropractors are not medical physicians or medical providers, so they need to hire a medical provider to offer medical treatment in their offices.

Years ago, chiropractors discovered that if they hired a genuine medical provider, such as a nurse practitioner (NP), physician assistant (PA), or an actual medical doctor (MD/DO), even just part-time for one day a week, they could effectively operate like a de facto medical office and offer genuine medical treatments instead of only chiropractic adjustments and related work.

In most states, medications, medical therapies, medical procedures, and medical treatments are outside the scope of a chiropractor's license. So, with a part-time medical provider on staff, a chiropractor can now offer all sorts of medical treatments for which they normally are prohibited from engaging in.

So, how did chiropractors get so heavy in the stem cell market when they aren't even allowed to prescribe that treatment or perform the injections?

The short answer is that it was a new, high-end, medical procedure that actually worked well to relieve pain and, most importantly, it could be administered by a part-time medical provider who came into the office once a week to perform all the procedures that the chiropractor sold to their patients during the week.

With an NP who comes once or twice a week, you can offer all these treatments and schedule them all on the day the NP is on site and operate like a medical office in the eyes of the patient, and in many cases these offices go the extra mile and remove "chiropractic" from the office name to enhance the medical aspect of the office.

A chiropractic office that employs a medical provider is usually called an "integrated chiropractic office," or simply an "integrated office" for short. This model has been very common for the last couple of decades.

In fact, there are whole consulting companies dedicated specifically to coaching chiropractors to appear like medical offices in the market, using this term "integrated medical office," where the intent is to rename your practice to something that doesn't include the term "chiropractor" in the title.

I've seen dozens of chiropractic offices change their names under these consultant groups' instructions. I've asked several of them why they changed the name and removed any reference to chiropractic services and the answers are that they want patients to see them as genuine medical offices with medical treatments, not just chiropractic services, even though the majority of the time the office is open there may not be a medical provider on site at all.

There's nothing wrong with a nurse practitioner working in a chiropractic office in this way, except when it becomes confusing to the patient about who is practicing medicine or who is the medical authority in the office.

A chiropractor is not a medical authority over a genuine medical provider like an NP, PA, or MD/DO, so if a patient is confused about this, it creates problems, yet it's that state of confusion that many chiropractors have counted on in order to sell high-dollar stem cell treatments for years.

Many states are starting to look at this model because if the chiropractor pays the salary of the medical provider, then the medical provider may be incentivized to perform medical services under the direction of the chiropractor, which they are not allowed to do because medical therapies are outside the scope of a chiropractor, and chiropractors are not allowed to dictate the course of medical care to a medical provider.

You can see how this is also confusing for medical providers employed by chiropractors. I've been in many of these offices and I've seen some that kept the appropriate line of authority in place, which is great and perfectly legitimate. I've also seen offices where the chiropractor operated like a medical doctor, wore a white coat, presented themselves like a medical physician, and discussed medical treatments with the patient, and of course sold expensive stem cell treatments.

Now take that environment of selling patients high-dollar stem cell treatments that aren't really stem cell treatments and you have a recipe for consumer fraud. This is what ultimately created the problems we saw in the stem cell treatment market several years ago, leading to wide-scale industry restrictions.

About ten years ago, as of this writing, one company in particular coached hundreds of chiropractic offices on selling high-dollar stem cell treatments. They advertised heavily and made a lot of promises.

One of the popular phrases was "one-and-done," indicating that you only need one injection and the stem cells would heal your tissues and that's all you would ever need. It doesn't work that way with these products. The underlying condition the patient has is still there. These injections help but don't cure anything.

This was a huge problem that ultimately led the FDA and the FTC to crack down on unscrupulous offices making all sorts of claims and charging obscene amounts of money to "cure" medical problems using products that aren't actually stem cells.

I'm all about innovation and creativity, and if all this somehow actually helped advance stem cell medicine, I wouldn't complain. But it didn't advance the field, it damaged the reputation of the field and even drove Google and Facebook to ban ads for stem cell therapies under pressure from government regulators ... yes, even for genuine stem cell therapies in legitimate offices, so it hurt everyone and set the whole industry back.

OK, I know I'm probably going a little too deep on this topic, but it's very important to understand this in terms of the condition of the stem cell market in the US because there's a reason you can only get certain types of stem cell therapy here in the US versus what's available around the world. BUT we are moving on in the world of stem cells to bigger and better things.

I just want those reading this to understand that history because I still get this question from people all the time: what's the deal with chiropractors and stem cells? Now you know a little about that.

**Will's Industry Insight #8:**
*Dose and concentration are everything! A quick note here on dosing, aka cell concentration. Standardization is the key ingredient in the future success of stem cell treatment.*

*Some companies have been compiling excellent documentation on the standardization of genuine stem cell and platelet-rich plasma (PRP) therapies in the world. And guess what the secret ingredient is for healing success? Dosing!*

*You have to concentrate the treatment high enough to produce enough stimulation to induce the in-situ cells and tissues to heal. If you don't concentrate the dose, you won't get the outcomes, and there are studies showing just how much concentration is needed to obtain those outcomes.*

We are well on our way to standardizing the regenerative medicine world by collecting all this excellent data on concentration and outcomes. For instance, most of the doctors who offer you a PRP injection in their office are only going to be able to concentrate it in a range of three to four times the concentration it naturally occurs in the blood.

What is the concentration needed to start seeing a huge difference in healing effect? Speaking to many providers and reviewing articles, 7x the normal concentration is the critical dose level to initiate efficacy, and 7x to 30x to get certain outcomes for certain tissues. This is all still in development and discovery with advances occurring all the time.

So, MOST doctors offering PRP are not even offering something that works on a significant therapeutic range. So, never make your choice based on price! The office down the street is going to claim to offer PRP cheaper, but they most likely aren't even in the same ballgame. Same for stem cells: you have to concentrate the dose to get the outcome.

That's why I love cultured expanded stem cell therapy, as I mentioned earlier. We can standardize this treatment and grow enough cells to concentrate the dose to create highly effective and successful outcomes. Dose and concentration are everything!

**Amniotic membrane stem cells:** The amniotic membrane is the actual sac that holds the fetus and fluid. It was one of the first tissues popularized for birth tissue stem cell use. The membrane is ideal because it has one of the lowest levels of immune markers on cell surfaces, nearly undetectable according to some research articles, so the risk of immune responses on recipients would be minimal to negligible.

**Amniotic membrane patches:** This happens to be an amazing wound care dressing for open wounds. It heals wounds and ulcers that are non-healing or difficult to treat. It's so good and so widely used that it's starting to become a standard of wound care treatment.

Most of these membranes are stripped of their cell content and dehydrated so it's not considered a stem cell product, but I've still heard it described to patients as a stem cell graft or a stem cell patch. It's not. It's just a dried piece of amniotic membrane with a lot of proteins that help tissues grow after being rehydrated on the wound. Still a great product for wound care though!

The amniotic membrane was used for numerous applications as a surgical dressing for burns and as an adjunctive tissue in surgical reconstruction of the oral cavity and bladder, and also for tympanoplasty, arthroplasty, repair of omphaloceles, and prevention of adhesions in pelvic and abdominal surgery.

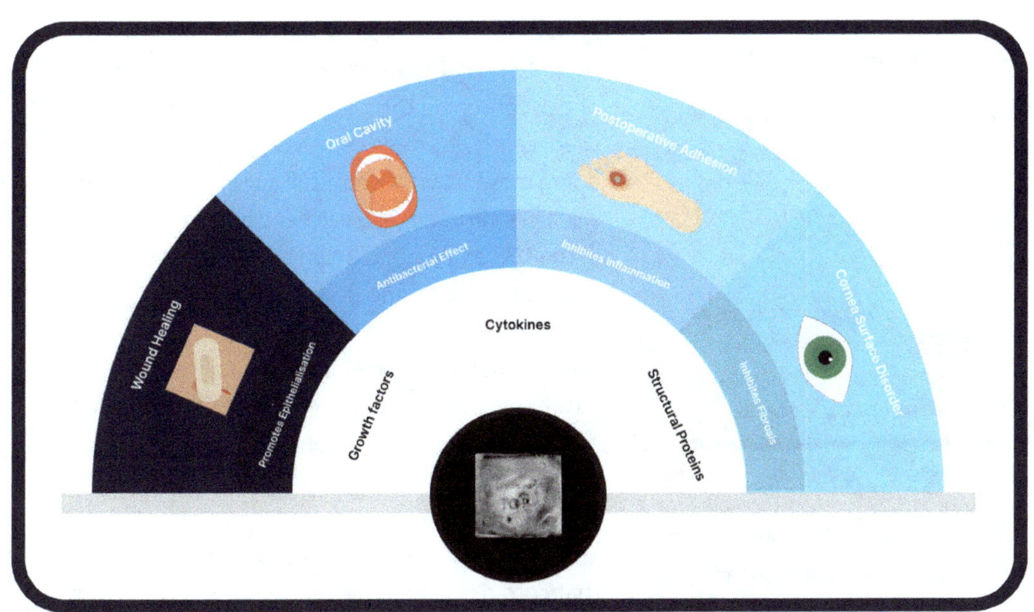


*Amniotic membrane components, characteristic, and applications*

*Data from: https://www.mdpi.com/2077-0375/11/12/941*

**Cord blood stem cells:** So, if I say blood, you say … hematopoietic. Correct! So, would these cells likely be used in your musculoskeletal treatment? There's a mix of cell types in cord blood, but ultimately cord blood stem cells for general regenerative medicine use and MSK use was heavily scrutinized a few years ago by the FDA and most of those operations were shut down quickly.

Labs were trying to find "the next best thing" to make and sell, but blood products are more complicated because they require blood type matching to be used, or they require more processing work to make them useful, so ultimately you only see cord blood stem cells in high-end medical research therapies like treating various cancers and organ damage.

It's a very exciting category of stem cells, but not the pathway of musculoskeletal treatment that I'm talking about here.

**Will's Industry Insight #9:**
*Cord tissue stem cells were popularized by a few companies looking to make something different from the more popular amniotic membrane products at the time, eight to 10 years ago.*

*What I know for certain, because I indirectly caused some of this required innovation, was that various researchers had non-compete contracts that prohibited them from working with amniotic membrane for any new company they worked for, so when those scientists left and worked for another company, or started their own labs, they couldn't work with amniotic membrane and instead worked with cord tissue.*

Cord tissue stem cells: This is the umbilical cord itself and all the tissue that makes it up. There's a good bit of cell content in this tissue that can be collected and used. Lately, it's been used as a great tissue source for doing mesenchymal stem cell culture and expansion work in international treatment programs, as the FDA in the US has clamped down on the injectable cord tissue product category.

Collecting the genuine mesenchymal cells out of this tissue for cell replication and expansion is probably going to be the most valuable aspect of this tissue category in the future.

They then had to create the industry perception that cord tissue was "better" or "newer" or "more advanced" than amniotic membrane, when there was no evidence of any superior quality other than that they could actually work with that tissue type under contract. (Just a little insight into why there are so many different product types on the market.)

Yes, I've been involved in conversations with a lot of these labs and companies when they were starting and I've been offered a lot of positions and partnerships and all sorts of things to come over and help these new ventures get off the ground. So I know some of these very intimate industry insights.

**Wharton's Jelly stem cells:** Wharton's Jelly is the gelatinous cushion that surrounds the vessels in the umbilical cord. It's rich in cell content and is a great tissue category to work with.

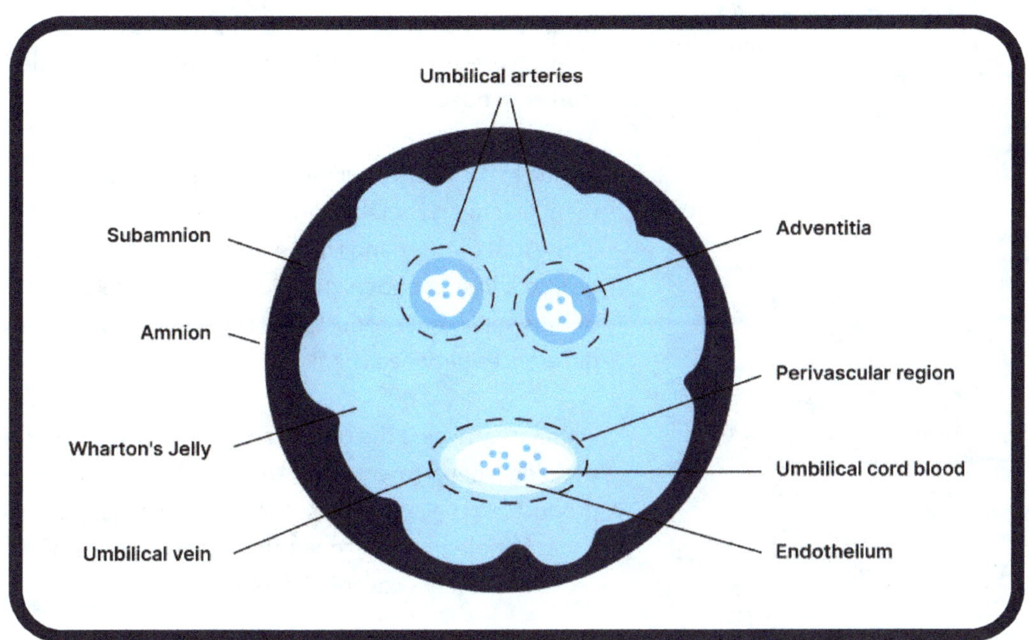


*Cross-sectional diagram of a human umbilical cord showing its anatomical compartments, including Wharton's jelly, as a source of stem cells.*

*Data: https://www.ncbi.nlm.nih.gov/pmc/articles/PMC3709752/*

Often, people use the terms "cord tissue" and "Wharton's Jelly" interchangeably, and although there are differences between them, they are both still great tissues for this industry. Again, we still can't do injections of products like these in the US anymore, but for a while, they were very popular. It's also commonly used in research and for cell culture and expansion.

**Placental stem cells:** The placenta is another source of cells, but for reasons of complexity I won't go into more detail, but it's still a tissue type you see used in some capacity.

Whew! That's a lot of info for a short run through. I could literally talk about each one of these categories all day. I used to do this all the time: spend endless hours researching and reading all about the cellular biology of all these tissues and spend hours on the phone explaining these details to doctors, labs, other biotech startup groups, and investors of all kinds.

I've even been on the phone with the CEOs and medical directors of some of the top four major commercial health insurance companies discussing the possibilities of adding these product types to their covered treatments. They loved the idea, but the market needed to be more established for them.

**Will's Industry Insight #10:**
*Minutiae of differences! Yep, as you can tell from the explanation above, there are a lot of minute details and differences between all these products. To make it even more complex, the FDA had categories to put all these products into and even those categories were nearly impossible for companies to interpret and distinguish.*

*Even today I hear of companies trying to make the case that their product is compliant in one category or another when, at the time of writing, the FDA has basically said none of these perinatal tissue products can be sold without now going through a drug trial, except amniotic membrane for wound covering. That's actually still a go and is reimbursable by Medicare and such, but everything else is non-compliant.*

Maybe in the future, but we're not there yet on reimbursement for these products. They were very interested though, and I had multiple calls with these groups and spent hours going over the fine details of these different products and the minutiae of differences between them.

I ultimately played the part of an expert witness to their legal departments over the risk of adding these products to their covered services because ultimately it was their legal department that vetoed the use of these products as covered benefits.

They loved hearing about the outcomes and cost efficiency of reducing surgeries and invasive procedures by using these products. I'm sure I'll talk to them again one day when the market is ready for it.

Even the companies making these products couldn't explain why their product wasn't the same as another or given the same status.

I had one company's executive team attempt to debate me on how their product was compliant, and I said to them, "I don't need to argue with you, I just need to see your FDA product compliance document – the paper that says your product is compliant under the category you're arguing about."

They couldn't do it, and they were really angry that I knew how to pin them down on this. In most of their sales conversations, they can simply obfuscate the details enough to where the doctor just stops asking questions and believes them.

I don't mince words with these groups anymore because they still damage and discredit the market. I tell them that just because they make a product following the guidelines of that category does not mean it's compliant in that category, and claiming to be compliant and collecting money from sales based on that claim is fraud.

That usually causes them all to pause for a few moments. I'm aiming for a real future in stem cell therapy so I can't suffer the fools who make us all look bad.

**Will's Industry Insight #11:**
*Stem cells are a dirty word! And it's because of all the charlatans out there! The regulations have now shifted to what you can't say, based on the abuse of all the common terms or words used to describe them.*

*Remember that what a doctor or chiropractor's office claims is stem cells that they pull out of the freezer is not stem cells, nor is it necessarily what they say it is. It's most likely a homogenized tissue injection that may contain a few viable stem cells at best, but it would be misleading to call it a stem cell injection, so regulations had to be enacted.*

Stem cells are a pretty easy term to regulate, so the FDA basically said anyone claiming to offer stem cell treatments or injections is in violation, so they simply track down all the ads and websites claiming stem cells.

Doctors and chiropractors would often change to another term to sell the same thing, so each new sales tactic resulted in another restricted word in the market. I've seen the progression of prohibited words keep going and going.

The latest advertisement I saw for a company selling products to doctors' offices called their product "a beneficial injection," using that term because no other word was allowed. So, the advertisement encouraged doctors to call and learn more about what this beneficial injection does for their patients.

"Our beneficial injection is the best beneficial injection on the market." You can see how bad it's gotten when these companies can't use "stem cells" or any other birth tissue name, can't use "regenerative medicine," can't say anything that indicates it's a biologic and are reduced to just calling it a "beneficial injection."

It's pretty comical in some respects, but speaks to how all the bad actors out there have ruined the market. Stem cells are a dirty word now, but my goal is to bring a real and regulated stem cell therapy to the US medical field.

# Chapter 2 - Non-Stem Cell Products

## *(Primarily used in the US market)*

So, what about non-stem cell products and treatments? There are a lot of them, and I'll run through them quickly. They are not the same thing as any of these above stem cell type therapies, but they do work and most likely some of these therapies will be the first to market as FDA-approved therapies that get covered by Medicare and commercial insurance companies.

**Acellular amniotic fluid – pure fluid:** Pure acellular amniotic fluid is amazing as a non-stem cell product. Its outcomes are excellent and it's a very simple product to make and standardize. There are no stem cells to worry about, so you don't have to count cells or worry about viability, which means you don't have to validate or prove cell counts and viability in the lab process.

And remember what I said before: most doctors say their outcomes are roughly as good or even better with pure fluid versus a cellular-based product. Remember all the reasons I mentioned before why a cellular product isn't what you think it is. Pure amniotic fluid is rich in growth factors and nutrients, and other beneficial things.

| Author, year (Ref) | Regenerated tissue | Treatment |
|---|---|---|
| **Kajiwara *et al.*, 2017, Kunisaki, 2018 (67, 69)** | Fetal | Congenital diaphragmatic hernia, abdominal wall defects, spinal bifida, and congenital heart |
| **Cipriani *et al.*, 2007 (68)** | Peripheral and central nervous | Neurodegenerative disease such as cerebral ischemia |
| **Di Baldassarre *et al* ., 2018 (70)** | Cardiac | Cardiomyoplasty |
| **Chun *et al.*, 2014 (71)** | Skeletal muscle | Duchenne muscular dystrophy |
| **Carraro *et al.*, 2008 (72)** | Lung | Lung-related disorders such as COVID-19 |
| **Morigi *et al.*, 2014 (73)** | Kidney | Acute ischemia-reperfusion and acute tubular necrosis |
| **Wang *et al.*, 2018 (74)** | Hepatic | Liver Abrosis |
| **Maraldi *et al.*, 2013 (75)** | Bone and cartilage | Extensive bone defects disease |
| **Chang *et al.*, 2018 (76)** | Ovarian | Ovarian dystrophy and fertility |
| **Gosemann *et al* ., 2012 (77)** | Inflammatory and autoimmune diseases | Graft-vs. host disease, inflammatory bowel disease, experimental autoimmune encephalomyelitis and systemic lupus erythematosus |

*Differentiation potential of human amniotic epithelial stem cells*

*Data from: https://www.ncbi.nlm.nih.gov/pmc/articles/PMC9596929/*

"Amniotic fluid is the perfect regenerative fluid mixture and the perfect regenerative medicine treatment because it's the biologically ideal mixture of components to support tissue growth and regeneration." – Will Bozeman.

Yep, I just quoted myself, but it's a true statement and I've been saying that for a decade now. The balance of growth factors and proteins is literally arranged in perfect ratios, so ultimately it would be the perfect fluid to use, no lab alteration required.

In fact, my most popular and successful product ever produced was the simplest version: pure amniotic fluid. We didn't alter it in any way; we simply filtered it for safety and left the concentrations exactly as is. This was the most successful regenerative product I've ever created in one of my biotech companies.

**PRP (PRFM, A2M, platelet lysate, and other PRP isolates):** Immediately I want to say that PRP is not all the same, and what your doctor calls PRP in their office may be vastly different from PRP in another office under different processing techniques. Dosing and concentration are everything when it comes to PRP. Keep that in mind as I explain the basics here.

Platelet-rich plasma was all the rage a couple of decades ago when a few high-end athletes mentioned getting PRP treatments for rapid recovery, which sparked a huge demand for PRP

| | |
|---|---|
| **Platelet-derived growth factor (PDGF)** | Enhances collagen synthesis, proliferation of bone cells, fibroblast chemotaxis and proliferative activity, macrophage activation |
| **Transforming growth factor ß (TGF-ß)** | Enhances synthesis of type I collagen, promotes angiogenesis, stimulates chemotaxis of immune cells, inhibits osteoclast formation and bone resorption |
| **Vascular endothelial growth factor (VEGF)** | Stimulates angiogenesis, migration and mitosis of endothelial cells, increases permeability of the vessels, stimulates chemotaxis of macrophages and neutrophils |
| **Epidermal growth factor (EGF)** | Stimulates cellular proliferation, differentiation of epithelial cells, promotes cytokine secretion by mesenchymal and epithelial cells |
| **Insulin-like growth factor (IGF)** | Promotes cell growth, differentiation, recruitment in bone, blood vessel, skin and other tissues, stimulates collagen synthesis together with PDGF |
| **Fibroblast growth factor (FGF)** | Promotes proliferation of mesenchymal cells, chondrocytes and osteoblasts, stimulates the growth and differentiation of chondrocytes and osteoblasts |

*Growth factors in PRP*

*Data from: https://www.ncbi.nlm.nih.gov/pmc/articles/PMC8046674/*

in the MSK field. Then a few celebrities and influencers promoted PRP for facials and hair regeneration and then suddenly it was all the rage in esthetics – and still is. PRP is created by drawing your blood, spinning it down and concentrating the plasma, drawing that back out, and then reinjecting it into the damaged tissue.

So, with all the processing techniques and processes out there, we can isolate almost any particular element out of your plasma and reinject that particular element instead of the whole plasma concoction.

This is an excellent advancement in regenerative medicine because all the studies show that different isolates of PRP are great at doing different things. So yeah, it can get complicated, and I won't go too far into the weeds on this, but I'll briefly mention the ones listed in the heading of this section.

PRP is platelet-rich plasma and is simply concentrated plasma. PRFM is platelet-rich fibrin matrix, which is simply PRP with a slightly different processing technique to make the mixture react differently and maybe more useful in some scenarios.

A2M is alpha-2-macroglobulin and is great at inhibiting cartilage deterioration (which occurs in patients with osteoarthritis) by binding up the reactive proteins in your joints that cause cartilage deterioration.

Platelet lysate is one of the many isolates of PRP that can create enhanced healing effects on specific tissues. Again, the dosage is everything with each of these versions of PRP. Yeah, it gets complicated and there is a lot of research going into these various treatments. It's actively being proven that the concentrations of these treatments are just as important as what's in them.

In some studies, a 4x concentration of PRP does nearly nothing, while a 7x concentration crosses the threshold into tissue activity, all with the same stuff, just more concentrated. So don't worry too much about the particulars at the moment, but know that when a doctor says "PRP," you want to know what exactly it is they are talking about.

**Exosomes or secretomes:** Exosomes are essentially the growth fluid used to grow stem cells in the lab. I create a plate of stem cells to grow in a dish and the nutrient-rich fluid the cells need is used by the cells and the leftover fluid has a lot of the beneficial elements of the stem cell growth process.

After the cells start growing, they produce little micro lipid packets of signaling proteins that are excreted from the cell, called exosomes – because they exit the cell – and they're little enclosed lipid bodies like bubbles, so "exit-body" or the more scientifically sounding "exosome" fits the description. They're also called secretomes because they're secreted from the cell.

If stem cells are an apple orchard, exosomes are the truck loads of apples leaving the orchard.

The first lab to bring exosomes to market years ago was an associate of mine, and we chatted a few times about the possibility of using this product. My first thought was that it could be a really interesting category, but it wasn't even a market category at all, so how would it be viewed by regulators and the medical community? I didn't know at all. I told them it sounded interesting, but it would be an unknown risk to bring it to market.

**Will's Industry Insight #12:**
*A company reached out to me a year after exosomes were in the market wanting my help on distribution and growth with their new "unique amniotic fluid" product line.*

*I asked them a few questions because amniotic fluid was an official, unique product designation, meaning it's not like anything else and the FDA recognizes this as a unique thing, which means you can't change it without calling it something else ... meaning your brand of amniotic fluid can't be "unique amniotic fluid" and still be compliant.*

*They told me they were growing amniotic fluid in the lab. I asked how they were doing that because amniotic fluid doesn't grow in labs. They said they were culturing stem cells and taking the growth fluid and making amniotic fluid because they were using amniotic membrane stem cells and that's what amniotic fluid was, right? Simple logic ... right? The fluid spins off from the amniotic membrane? You can see how complicated the definitions can be.*

Fast-forward a couple years and they were selling across the nation, and a dozen other groups were making their own exosome products. So, exosomes were all the hype for a few years and got a lot of negative attention, and, ultimately, you don't see them much anymore.

Exosomes are still around, but they got hammered by the FDA for misrepresentation because sales reps and companies were selling them under the wrong terms. They started out calling them stem cells like everything else, but when stem cells became a dirty word, they switched to calling exosomes "amniotic fluid." Why? Let me throw in a little Will's Industry Insight here to explain.

Keep in mind that I was on the phone with the top executives at this biotech company: the CEO, their Chief Medical Officer, their Chief Science Officer, and their Chief Sales Officer. They were the ones who were deciding how to educate their clients, doctors, on what this product was that they were selling.

I said, "What you're describing is not amniotic fluid, it's exosomes."

Long pause. "Yeah, we know it's actually exosomes, but," here are their own words and I wish I had recorded this, "it's too difficult to educate doctors on the nuances of different products, so we just call it amniotic fluid because they understand that and it's more acceptable to them."

So, there you have it: the reason for all the regulations and problems we've had in the regenerative medicine industry over the last five years. You can't call it what it isn't. So, after they got caught calling it the wrong thing, which I thoroughly warned them about, they were forced to change their description type to a new term, "amniotic derived fluid," which again, was all to avoid calling it what it actually was: exosomes.

All this was because it was too hard to explain exosomes and there were already major competitors in the market for exosomes and they wanted something unique that couldn't be replicated by competitors. So, this company thought they'd be clever and create a new market category, but the FDA moved all lab grown products into another classification later and that basically stopped everyone in their tracks on exosomes.

**Peptides:** This is an exciting new field of medicine with a lot of potential. Peptides are protein compound segments that are created to affect certain cellular responses. Stem cells are the orchard, exosomes are the apples, and peptides are the juice in the apples. Cells are looking for the signals from other cells to communicate and take action.

Peptides are great because they can be grown in the lab and all sorts of specific peptides can be isolated and grown in concentration. I believe there is exceptional biologic standardization potential with peptides, so I'm actively keeping an eye on peptides and looking forward to innovation in that field.

**Prolotherapy:** Prolotherapy is a dextrose sugar injection that agitates the tissues at the cellular level and creates a mild inflammation with a healing effect afterward, like doing an exfoliating scrub on your face to remove all the dead skin and the after-effect creates fine, smooth skin.

Some physicians wouldn't call prolotherapy a true regenerative medicine therapy in the same category as these other items above, but many do feel that it qualifies as a regenerative.

It's great of course, but you're not adding any regenerative elements to this process, you're simply agitating tissue to become mildly inflamed and then letting it heal back up. In short, it's simply creating a mild local tissue irritation through dextrose sugar crystals roughing up the cells and tissue and causing inflammation and mild tissue damage in that area for the cells to be agitated and triggered into healing.

I've talked to doctors who do consider it regenerative, but I've talked to a lot of doctors about this, and with all the better options out there, stem cells, PRP, and other options, it's hard to justify doing old-school prolotherapy except that it's so affordable because dextrose is really cheap, and the injections are very simple and easy.

That's the wrap-up on the general overview of regenerative medicine in the US. Keep in mind that by the time you read this, some of the things I mentioned may have new regulations and you may not find some of these options at all.

Now, let's talk about spinal stenosis and how regenerative medicine treatments are changing the entire treatment strategy for this condition. You have options, and stem cells for degenerative spine conditions may be exactly what you need!

# Chapter 3 - Introduction to Spinal Stenosis

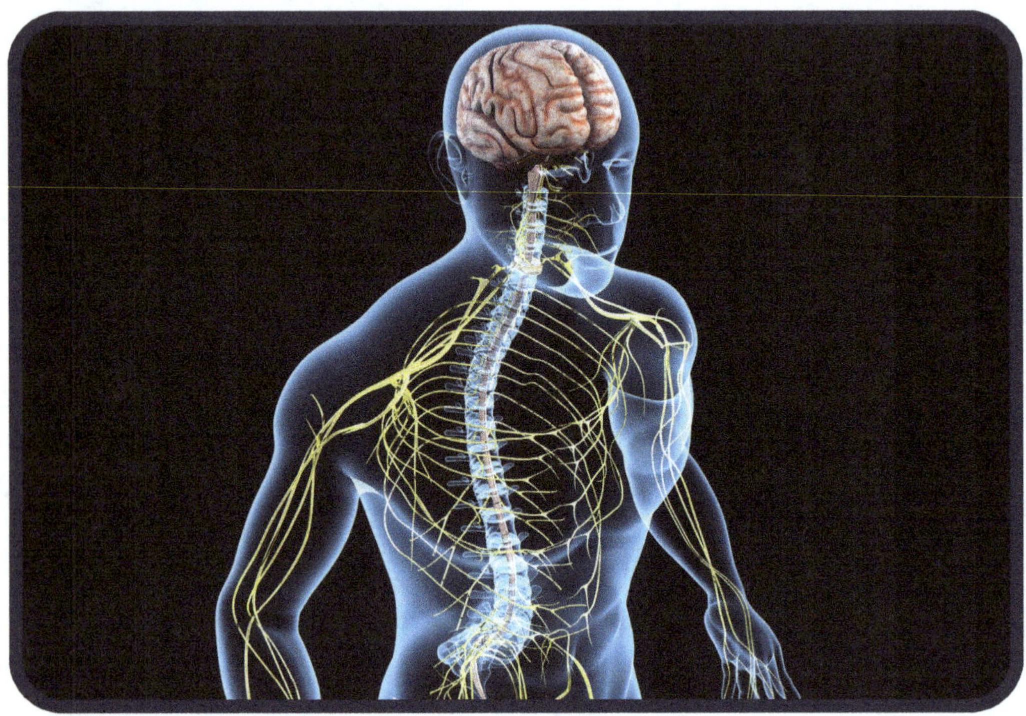

The spine houses 31 pairs of spinal nerves, which are responsible for connecting the different parts of the body and various organs to the central nervous system - or the nerves in the brain and spinal cord. These spinal nerves, which are located within a secure, sturdy passageway known as the spinal canal, transmit motor, sensory, and autonomic signals, which control touch sensation, muscle movements, and functions such as breathing, heartbeat, and digestion.

While the spinal canal does an excellent job of providing the spinal nerves with a safe and spacious case, certain health conditions and age-related degenerative changes can narrow this canal. The narrowing of the spinal canal can put excessive, undue pressure on the nerve roots, thus interfering with the normal transmission of nerve signals. This condition, which is estimated to affect 250,000-500,000 US residents, is known as spinal stenosis. (1)

Not everyone with spinal stenosis will experience symptoms immediately. However, if left unaddressed, this condition can lead to severe chronic pain, numbness, weakness, and, eventually, permanent nerve damage and disability.

What complicates this picture even further is the fact that, often, individuals with spinal stenosis resort to medications and doubtful treatments, which do very little to cure the disease and can cause severe side effects. Even worse, when damaged nerves and other components of the spine are damaged beyond repair, the only prospect left for millions of patients is invasive, painful, and highly risky spinal surgeries.

Fortunately, thanks to the advances in stem cell therapies I have unveiled in the sections above, there is a lot that can be done to help you manage your symptoms and regain the function of your spine and nerves. In the following chapters, I'll delve into the nature, causes, risk factors, and outlook of spinal stenosis, and I'll take you through the treatments made available by the advances in stem cell technologies.

# History and Significance of Spinal Stenosis

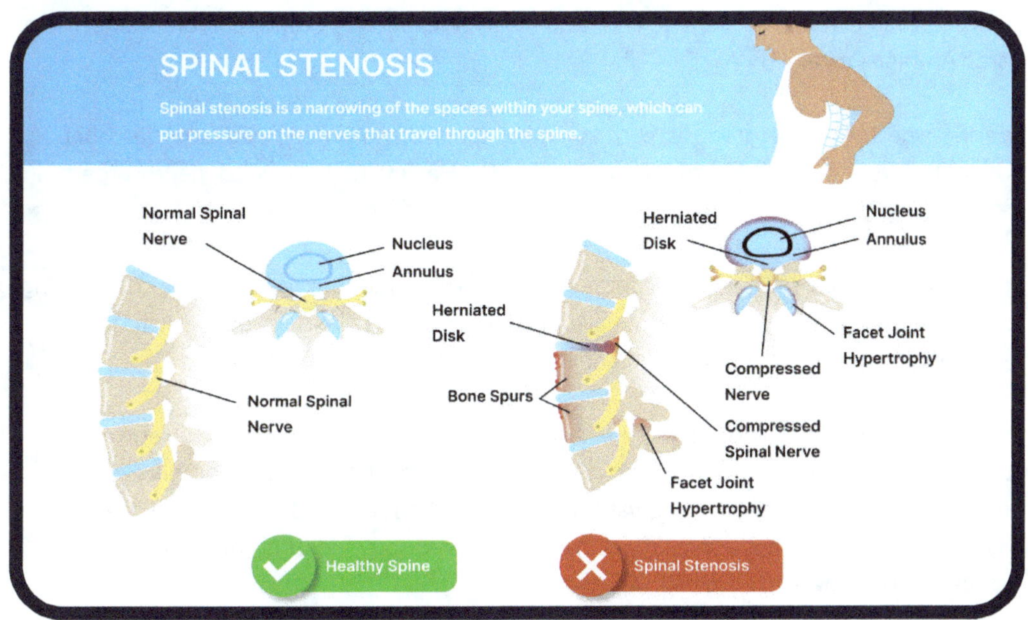

Degenerative changes occur in most people's spines by the time they are 50 - and one of the most common changes is the narrowing of the spinal canal, which leads to spinal stenosis. As the global population continues to age, this condition, among other chronic pain disorders affecting the spine, is increasing in prevalence and becoming a major healthcare concern.

To aggravate this picture is the fact that around 40% of patients with painful conditions affecting the lower spine take opioids as part of their treatments.(2) Not only are these prescriptions inefficient in modifying the disease, but they can also lead to severe side effects, including increased tolerance, addiction, overdose, and death.

Ultimately, opioids prescribed for orthopedic problems and chronic pain conditions are significantly fueling the opioid epidemics that are still raging across the nation.

Having a better understanding of the history, prevalence, and prognosis of spinal stenosis can help you make well-informed decisions about your chosen line of treatment and avoid the side effects of medications and surgery. Let's look at these aspects below.

## First Cases

The history of spinal stenosis takes us back to Ancient Egypt when the first cases of this condition were documented. However, it wasn't until 1803 that a modern description of spinal stenosis became available to the scientific community, crafted by French anatomist and doctor Baron Antoine Portal. (3)

Specific aspects of spinal stenosis, such as lumbar spinal stenosis (LSS) were only described during the 1900s, with formal definitions credited to Henk Verbiest, a Dutch neurosurgeon, in 1954. (4)

Following Verbiest's definition, LSS became recognized as a serious medical issue contributing to physical disability. Researchers like Porter and his colleagues later linked the symptoms of persistent back pain and weakness to a shrinking spinal canal. (4)

In the 1990s, a research trio - Johnsson, Rosén, and Udén - conducted a study on untreated spinal stenosis patients. Their research offered key insights on the possible progression, prognosis, and treatment of LSS. It was found that most patients (70%) reported little to no change in their symptoms, a small number (15%) showed some deterioration, and, rarely, neurological decline also occurred. (4)

These studies opened the way to successful surgical treatments for spinal stenosis, though, at first, these were primarily based on surgeons' subjective evaluations. Between the late 19th century and the beginning of the 20th century, the first successful spinal fusion surgery was performed to prevent progressive deformities linked to spinal stenosis, such as Pott's disease (i.e. tuberculosis of the spine).

At the same time, laminectomy emerged as a surgical option to treat spinal stenosis due to cauda equina syndrome.

Over the past two centuries, advancements in technologies, research, and equipment have opened the way to a greater range of viable treatment options. Nonetheless, today, the US Social Security Act acknowledges spinal stenosis as a debilitating, disability-causing condition, especially when it affects the lower spine. (5)

## Vulnerability

Spinal stenosis can affect anyone, at any stage of life. However, the most vulnerable demographic is adults aged 50 and over. This condition is also more common among females than males.

This age-related vulnerability is due to degenerative changes that typically occur in the spine as we age. These may include the increased propensity to herniated and bulging disks, as well as chronic musculoskeletal conditions like arthritis. These disorders can change the structure of the spinal canal, leading to abnormal narrowing of this structure and, in turn, spinal stenosis.

High-impact athletes who perform forceful movements that put excessive stress on the spine can also be at risk of overuse-related changes in the spinal canal.

Additionally, those with a family history of spinal stenosis or who are born with abnormalities (e.g. thinner cartilage) may be more likely to develop spinal stenosis during their lifetimes. In the following sections, I'll explain the causes and risk factors of spinal stenosis in more detail.

## Levels of Occurrence

Spinal stenosis is a relatively common condition that tends to mostly affect aging adults.

According to a review conducted using the Medicare dataset, nearly a third of Medicare enrollees had some form of spine degeneration. (6) Spinal stenosis was found to be the third most common disorder, after disc degeneration and osteoporosis, with a mean prevalence among adults aged 65-85+ of 4.5%.

However, this condition affected over 6% of those aged between 70 and 80, and it was far more common among females. Other forms of spine degeneration affecting the elderly include spine curvature, spondylitis, disc degeneration, osteoporosis, and diffuse idiopathic skeletal hyperostosis (DISH).

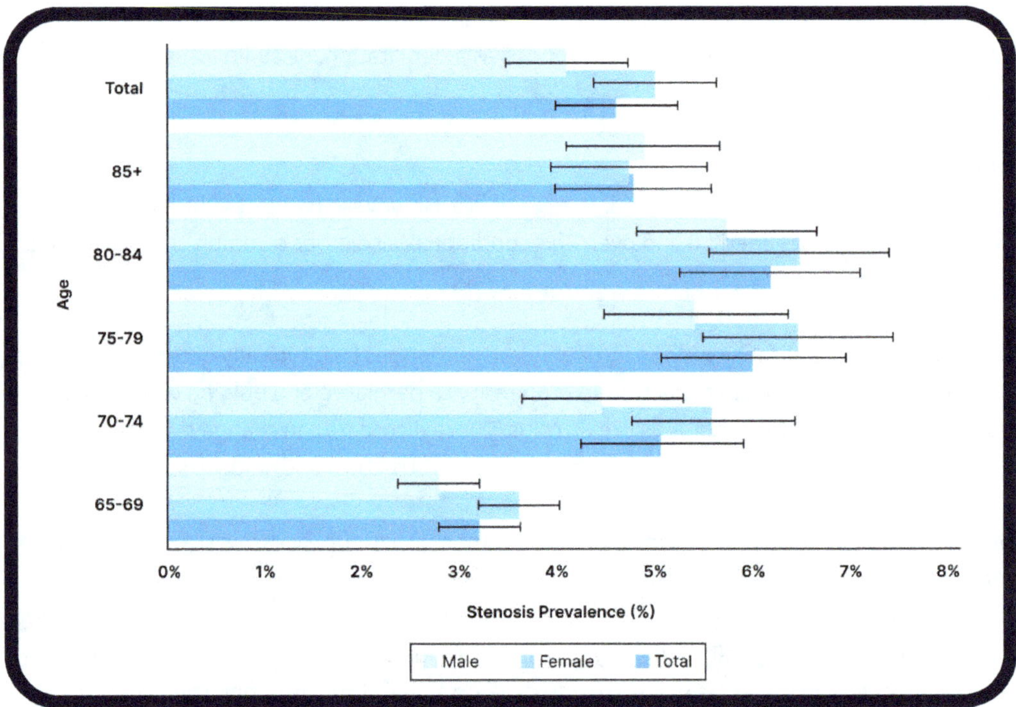


*Prevalence of spine degeneration diagnoses by age group*

*Data from: https://www.ncbi.nlm.nih.gov/pmc/articles/PMC7940625/*

It is also important to note that the prevalence of spine degeneration types is far greater among those diagnosed with obesity. In particular, spinal stenosis was two to three times more prevalent in obese patients.

Due to the increasing rates of obesity and the aging of the population, spinal stenosis and other degenerative changes of the spine are more frequently diagnosed today than in the past. (7) Between 2005 and 2017, the prevalence of spine degeneration increased from 24% to 30% among the elderly.

## Impact

When spinal stenosis is left untreated, it can become a long-term condition that affects all aspects of your life. Due to chronic pain, reduced mobility, weakness, and numbness, you may find it more challenging to complete daily tasks.

Not only can this lead to frustration and anxiety, but it can also increase the risk of social withdrawal and mental health conditions like depression. According to a 2021 review of 24 studies, nearly 31% of people with degenerative spine disease - 24% of those with lumbar spine stenosis - showed clinical symptoms of depression. (8)

Besides leading to mental health conditions, degenerative spine conditions may also impact your employability and productivity. Low back pain, which may be caused by lumbar spinal stenosis, is widely considered one of the leading causes of missed work days and years lived with disability - as well as the most common form of chronic pain - in the US and worldwide.

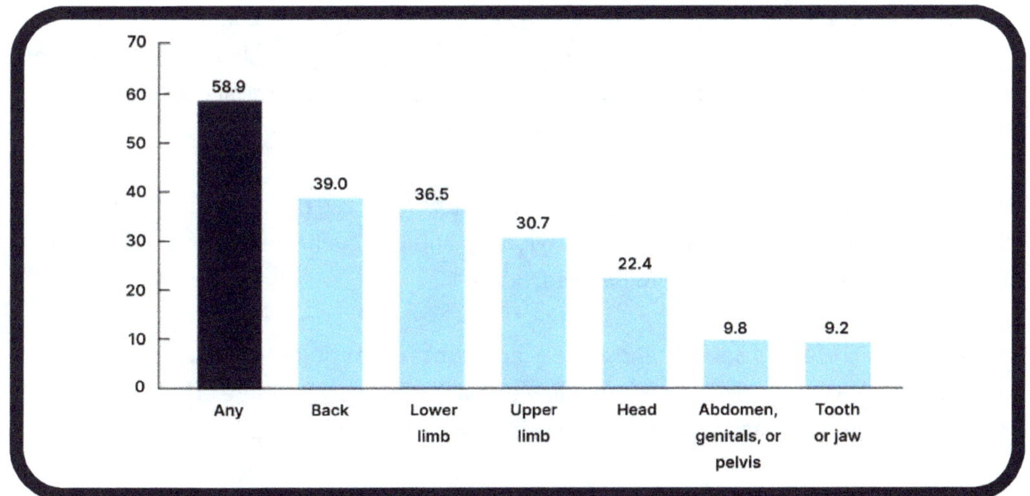


*Percentage of adults aged 18 and over with any pain and pain by body region*

*Data from: https://www.cdc.gov/nchs/products/databriefs/db415.htm*

Another impactful aspect of living with spinal stenosis is cost, both direct and indirect, associated with this condition. Estimates show that managing spinal stenosis without surgery (i.e. with medication, at-home remedies, and therapies such as massage therapy and physiotherapy) costs an average of $59,071 over two years. (9)

The same study shows that treating this condition with surgery may be able to lower these costs and reduce mortality rates. However, this choice may expose patients to health risks, lengthy rehabilitation times, and a significant financial burden associated with covering the costs of surgery.

When it comes to reducing the impact of spinal stenosis, significant emphasis is put on prevention and prompt treatment. Addressing this condition as soon as the first symptoms manifest themselves is one of the most efficient strategies for finding an adequate line of treatment and reducing the risk of complications.

Nonetheless, thanks to today's advances in regenerative orthopedic medicine, new, efficient, and non-invasive treatment alternatives have become available.

**Future**

With the aging of the population and the rising rates of obesity, spinal stenosis is expected to become more prevalent. Given its chronic and long-term nature, this condition brings a pressing need to develop innovative treatment solutions. Currently, as I'll explain later in this book, treatment methods mostly revolve around injections, pharmaceutical management, physiotherapy, or in more serious cases, invasive surgery.

However, each of these treatments has its limitations. Chronic use of pharmaceuticals can lead to side effects, and surgery often comes with long, painful recovery periods. It is easy to see that there's a medical gap waiting to be filled.

Fortunately, the future of spinal stenosis treatment looks promising and open to innovation. Driven by necessity, new medical technologies are paving the way for more efficient, non-invasive, and non-pharmaceutical treatments - including stem cell therapies.

These therapies do more than simply address the symptoms of spinal stenosis. They leverage the body's self-healing capabilities to reverse disease, lay the foundation of long-term health, and magnify each patient's quality of life.

# Experiencing Spinal Stenosis

As I explained above, spinal stenosis occurs when there is an abnormal narrowing of the spinal canal, or the "passageway" that houses the nerves of the spinal cord - a bundle of nerves that come out of the base of the brain, runs down the center of the spine, and splits off to innervate several areas of the body.

Spinal stenosis is a medical term derived from Greek origins: "Stenosis," meaning narrowing, and "spinal," pertaining to the spine.

This abnormal narrowing - or, simply, stenosis - can affect any passage, organ, or structure in the body with a tubular shape. When the diameter of the tube is reduced, dysfunctions take place.

In the case of spinal stenosis, this abnormal narrowing can affect one or more areas of the spine:

- The spinal canal - the canal composed of the hollow spaces in the center of each spinal bone (vertebrae), stacked up
- The spaces in the spinal canal from which the nerve roots branch out of the spinal cord
- The spaces between the vertebrae, which are used by the nerves to leave the spine and travel to other areas of the body

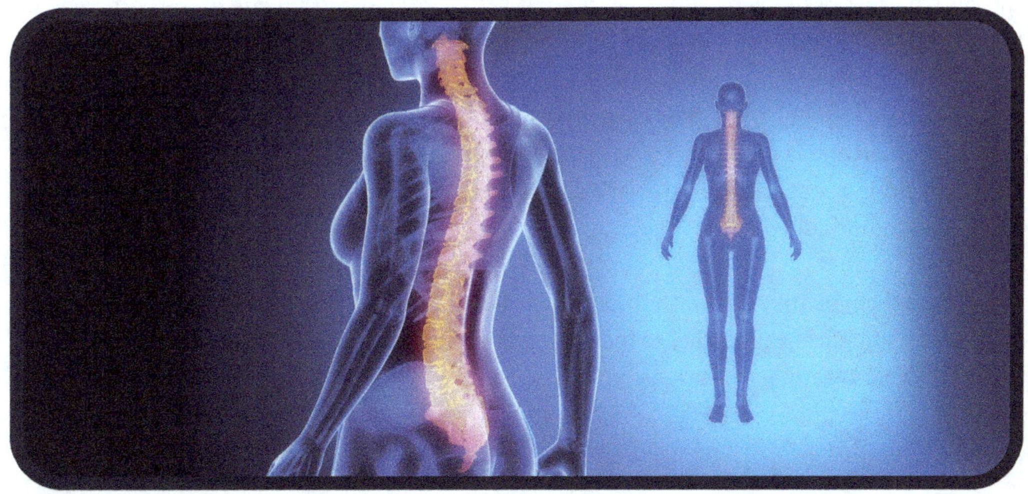

Spending on what structures of the spine are affected by the abnormal narrowing of the spinal canal, you may have to deal with the consequences of two different complications:

- **Radiculopathy.** Radiculopathy occurs when the nerve roots are pinched in the area where they exit the spinal cord. Radiculopathy is commonly associated with numbness, tingling, and loss of sensation in the areas regulated by the compressed nerves.
- **Myelopathy.** Myelopathy is a condition that occurs when the spinal cord itself is compressed. Myelopathy leads to more serious symptoms, including severe pain, coordination and balance issues, loss of function, and loss of bladder and bowel control. Myelopathy can also lead to a common complication of spinal stenosis: neurogenic claudication. (10)

  This complication causes pain, weakness, or tingling in your lower back and legs. This usually occurs when you're standing or walking, due to the pressure applied on your spinal nerves.

  One of the most common forms of myelopathy is cervical spondylotic myelopathy (CSM), a neurologic condition that develops over time when spinal stenosis results in compression of the cord. While this is considered to be the most common form of spinal cord injury in adults, its diagnosis is often delayed.

Spinal stenosis is a degenerative condition. This means that, at first, you may not notice much more than mild discomfort or back pain. However, over time, this disorder can translate into chronic pain, loss of mobility, and diminished daily functioning, mostly due to the narrowing of the spinal canal that presses on your nerves.

What's more, these degenerative changes in the spine are often caused by another condition, such as osteoarthritis or a slipped disc. In particular, results from a 2012 study specify that "Spinal stenosis is associated with a very substantial burden of illness that is compounded by associated comorbidities." (11)

This means that you may deal with the symptoms of more than one chronic condition at a time, which impacts your ability to manage your symptoms, hinders your recovery, and influences your treatment decisions.

In your daily life, you may find that spinal stenosis makes accomplishing routine tasks increasingly challenging. Simple chores like grocery shopping or taking a walk may become uphill battles, mostly due to discomfort or pain. Additionally, the pain can make movement undesirable, thus affecting your ability to remain active and lead a healthy lifestyle.

The constant discomfort might also affect your sleep. Quality rest becomes elusive, leaving you fatigued and irritable during the day, increasing your levels of stress, and adding fuel to the fire that is systemic inflammation.

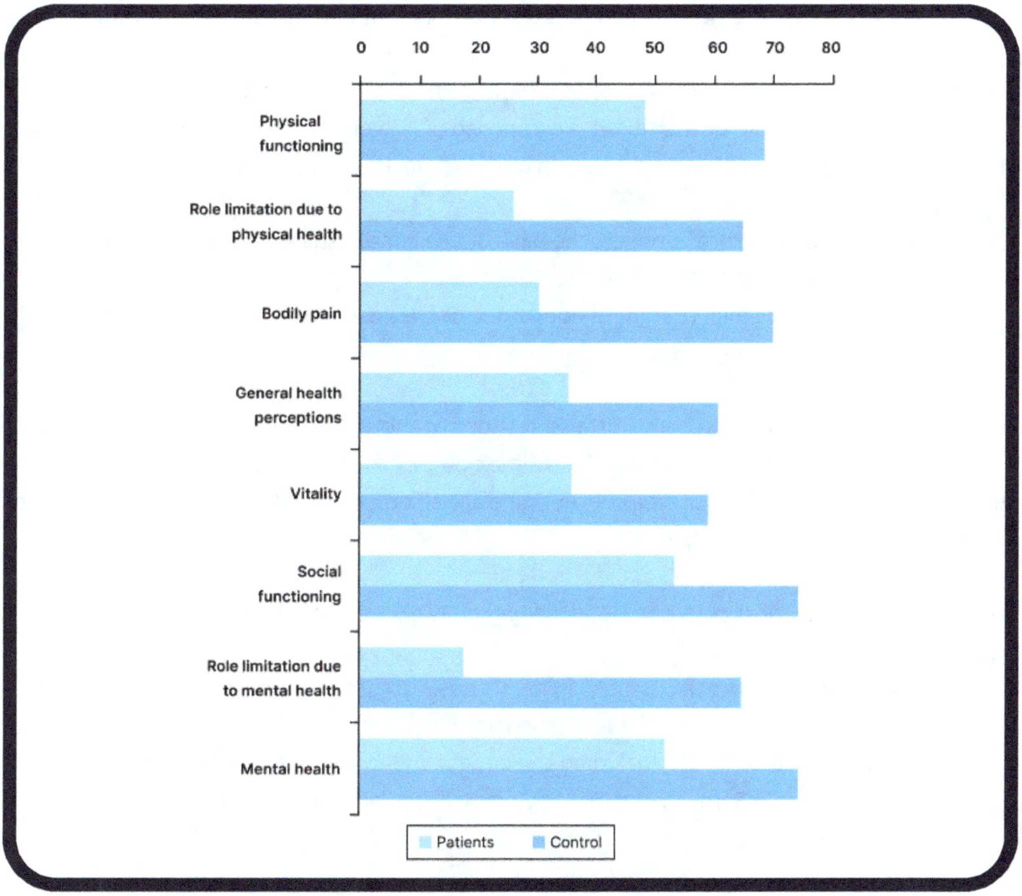

*Comparison between quality of life in patients with chronic low back pain for 3 months or longer and healthy control participants. The patients suffering from low back pain reported lower scores in all criteria.*

*Data from: https://pubmed.ncbi.nlm.nih.gov/25006368/*



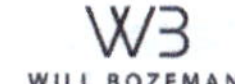

To prevent the catastrophic consequences that spinal stenosis can have on your mental and physical well-being, it is important to pinpoint its early symptoms and seek adequate treatment. Below, I'll explore the telltale signs that you may be battling degenerative changes in the spine.

## Symptoms

The spine is composed of different sections that work together to enable movements, protect you from injury, and support the body. The four main regions of the spine are:

- **Cervical spine.** The neck region of the spine. It is composed of seven vertebrae (C1-C7).
- **Thoracic spine.** The middle section of your spine, which runs from the base of your neck to the bottom of the ribs. It is composed of 12 vertebrae (Th1-Th12).
- **Lumbar spine.** The lower back region of the spine. It is composed of five vertebrae (L1-L5).
- **Sacrum.** This structure connects the base of the lumbar spine to the pelvis. It is composed of three bones fused together.
- **Coccyx.** This is a small triangle-shaped bone at the base of the spine. It is composed of four bones fused together.

While spinal stenosis can affect any of these sections of the spine, it most commonly develops in the lumbar spine and cervical spine. The thoracic part of the spine may also be affected, but this is rare. Depending on what areas of the spine are affected by stenosis, you may experience certain symptoms, in specific areas.

Below, I'll look at the most common signs that you may have spinal stenosis.

- **Lumbar spinal stenosis.** Lumbar spinal stenosis occurs when the narrowing of the spinal canal affects the lower (lumbar) spine. It tends to affect the nerves that innervate the lower body, including the largest and longest nerve in the body - the sciatic nerve. (12) Some of the most common symptoms of this condition include:
    - Pain in the lower back
    - Pain that begins in the buttocks and radiates down to the leg and may also extend to the foot
    - A heavy feeling in the legs, as well as weakness and involuntary muscle movements, such as cramps or spasms

- Numbness, tingling, and "pins and needles" sensations, which are known as paresthesia, a complication of nerve damage. It may affect your buttocks, legs, or feet.
- Pain that intensifies when standing for long periods of time or walking (especially when walking downhill). This type of pain may also ease down when you are leaning forward - which relieves the pressure on the spine - sit, or walk uphill.

- **Cervical spinal stenosis.** Cervical spinal stenosis occurs in the first section of the spine, around the neck area or the base of the skull. In this case, you are likely to experience symptoms anywhere below the point of compression of the nerve. Depending on what nerves are affected, you may experience the following symptoms:
    - Neck pain
    - Numbness and tingling, affecting the arm, hand, leg, or foot
    - Weakness in the arm, hand, leg, or foot
    - Clumsiness and loss of grip strength
    - Balance and coordination problems
    - Impaired hand function, such as having trouble writing or buttoning clothes

In any case, spinal stenosis is characterized by pain, numbness, tingling, and weakness. The intensity, nature, and location of these symptoms may vary from one person to another. For example, some describe the pain as a dull ache or tenderness, while others experience burning, electric shock-like sensations. While the pain may come and go, it tends to worsen over time.

In severe cases (e.g. if the entire spinal cord is compressed), or if left untreated, spinal stenosis can also lead to life-disrupting complications. These include:

- Loss of bladder or bowel control (incontinence)
- Sexual dysfunction due to nerve damage, such as erectile dysfunction and anorgasmia
- Partial or complete leg paralysis

## Demographics at Risk

Spinal stenosis can affect anyone, at any age. However, certain individuals are at a higher risk of developing this disease.

Studies have shown that five in 1000 people over the age of 50 are likely to get spinal stenosis. What's more, the chances of developing those disorders increase with age.

Nonetheless, younger people who are born with a narrow spinal canal, have reported injuries to the spine, or regularly place their spine under undue stress may also be at risk of spinal stenosis.

The typical patient showing signs of spinal stenosis is either an aging adult - more commonly female - with degenerative changes of the spine or younger people involved in sports and professional activities that overly stress the spine.

| Type of LSS | Relative (≤ 12 mm) (N=191) | | Absolute (≤ 10 mm) (N=191) | |
|---|---|---|---|---|
| | N | % (95% CI) | N | % (95% CI) |
| Congenital | 9 | 4.71% (2.18-8.76%) | 5 | 2.62% (0.86-6.00%) |
| Acquired | 14 | 22.50% (16.80-29.10%) | 14 | 7.30% (4.07-11.99%) |
| Any Type | 45 | 23.60 (17.73-30.23%) | 16 | 8.40% (4.86-13.25%) |

***Prevalence of congenital and acquired lumbar spinal stenosis in the population-based sample.***

*Data from: https://www.ncbi.nlm.nih.gov/pmc/articles/PMC3775665/*

According to studies, lumbar spinal stenosis is one of the most commonly diagnosed and treated pathologic conditions affecting the spine. It is estimated that congenital stenosis occurs in up to 7% of the population, while a degenerative form of the disease affects up to a third of adults. (13) There are also significant geographical variations in the prevalence of degenerative spine disease.

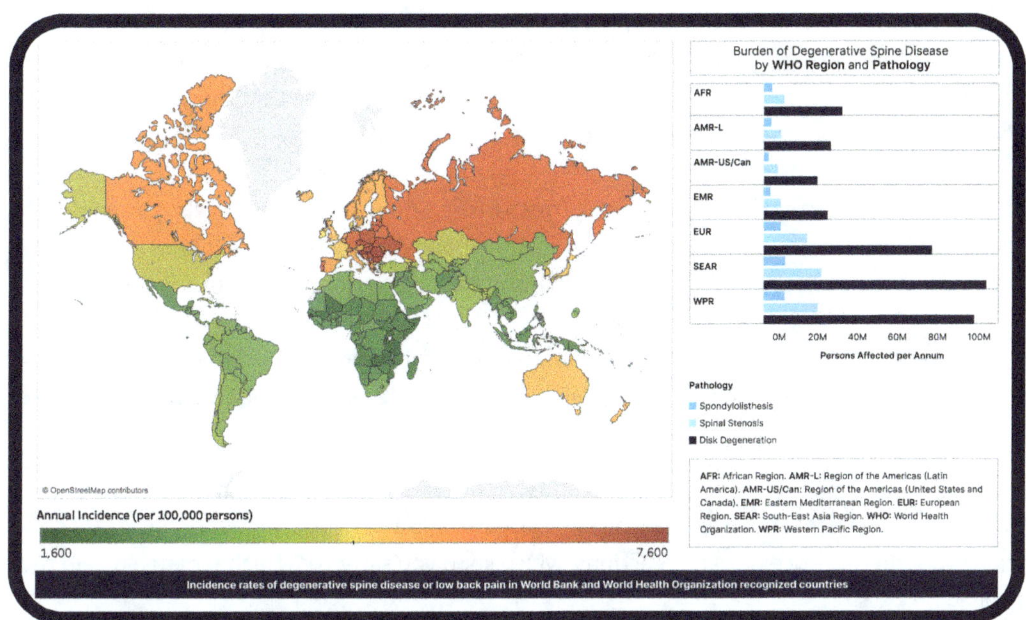


*Incidence rates of degenerative spine disease or low back pain in World Bank and World Health Organization recognized countries.*

*Data from: https://journals.sagepub.com/doi/10.1177/2192568218770769*

# Difference Between Chronic and Acute Spinal Stenosis

As I've explained above, spinal stenosis can have catastrophic consequences on your mental and physical health, especially if not adequately addressed. But not all forms of spinal stenosis are equal - nor do they have the same causes, prognosis, or impact.

Because of this, it is crucial to understand whether the pain you are experiencing is acute or chronic. In the sections below, I'll explore the differences between acute and chronic spinal stenosis, and I'll highlight why it is important to keep this difference in mind.

## Chronic vs Acute Spinal Stenosis: An Overview

To understand the difference between chronic and acute spinal stenosis, I'll take a step back and explain the difference between acute and chronic pain.



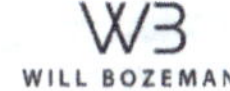

Simply, pain is a "language" your body uses to signify harm or danger, and it helps keep your body safe from further injury. Think, for example, of when you burn your hand or touch something painful - you'll experience a painful sensation and a reflex that causes you to bring your body away from the source of danger.

These signals are carried by the complex infrastructure of nerves and chemicals (hormones) across the body. These same agents also trigger an inflammatory response in the event of injury, which is necessary to contain the damage and kick-start the body's healing process.

This concept, although simple on the surface, can become complex when looking at the fact that not all types of pain are created equally. Here's the difference between chronic and acute pain:

- **Acute pain**

Acute pain is the consequence of an injury or disease. It is a biological response necessary to trigger a series of processes and reactions, which keep you safe from further harm and aid the healing process.

Here's how acute pain occurs: a dangerous or painful agent activates the sympathetic nervous system and the nerve endings around the damaged, diseased, or injured area - which are known as nociceptors - send information to the brain. As your brain senses the pain, it begins to organize a response to the attacker.

Acute pain can be caused by a wide range of health events, such as broken bones, surgery, dental work, ligament tears, burns, cuts, and even childbirth. In the case of spinal stenosis, you may experience acute pain if the narrowing of the spine is caused by a sudden or traumatic injury - such as a spinal injury or disc herniation.

It is important to keep in mind that acute pain is self-limited. This means that, once the underlying injury is treated, it will go away on its own and won't lead to further damage.

Think, for example, of a fracture in the vertebrae. Once adequately treated, the space in the spinal canal is restored and the symptoms of spinal stenosis will subside. Acute pain usually lasts less than six months. While you are undergoing treatment for the cause of pain, you may take advantage of medications that stop nociceptive signals, which prevent you from experiencing pain.

- **Chronic pain**

Chronic pain represents a different clinical entity compared to acute pain. It tends to last longer than six months and persists far longer after the injury or disease (which activates the nociceptors) has healed. What's more, in most cases, chronic pain isn't triggered by a health event, such as trauma or illness.

Instead, it tends to arise from a combination of psychological, lifestyle, and environmental factors. Another difference is that chronic pain does not serve a biological purpose and does not have an identifiable end-point.

If you suffer from chronic back pain, the nervous system remains active for days on end and keeps sending pain signals to the brain, even though there is no injury or disease.

In response to pain, the brain increases the levels of inflammation which, when uncontrolled, can lead to permanent damage of various musculoskeletal components, including nerves (which leads to neuropathy), bones, ligaments, and cartilage.

New theories are now offering an alternative explanation for chronic pain. (14) Research is exploring the role of systemic inflammation in the development of chronic diseases (e.g. diabetes and cardiovascular disease), as well as chronic pain and reduced longevity.

When systemic inflammation is at the root of your chronic back pain, you may also experience chronic fatigue, muscle tension, and a decline in mental health due to social isolation, inactivity, anxiety, and depression.

Spinal stenosis can occur due to a sudden trauma, injury, or disease. However, if it is not properly addressed - or badly treated - you may find yourself dealing with long-lasting changes in the spine. These, in turn, can lead to the permanent narrowing of the spinal canal, which leads to chronic pain.

In the next few chapters of this book, I'll take you through the treatment options available to manage chronic pain and tackle the systemic inflammation at the root of your disease.

However, for now, it is crucial to keep in mind that what truly complicates the clinical picture of many patients suffering from chronic pain is their assumption that their condition can't be cured.

This is due to difficulties in adequately diagnosing chronic pain, as well as the inadequate approach by physicians, and problems with healthcare insurance coverages, such as "fail-first" policies.

Below, I'll explain the causes and risk factors of spinal stenosis, and I'll discuss the importance of preventing your condition from degenerating from acute to chronic.

## Causes of Spinal Stenosis

Spinal stenosis can arise from a combination of probable and possible contributors. As we have seen above, the degenerative changes of the spine that occur with age are certainly the main culprit for the emergence of this condition. Nonetheless, it is possible to develop an abnormal narrowing of the spinal canal due to several other reasons.

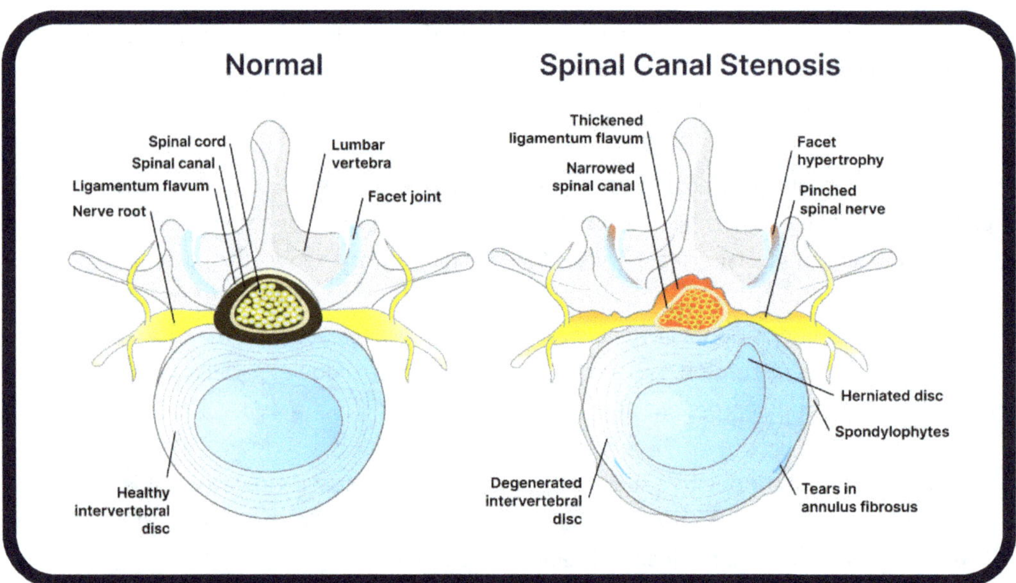


Additionally, it is important to keep in mind that spinal stenosis can be acquired (developing any time after birth) or congenital (developing from birth). These two conditions can have different causes and triggering factors. I'll cover the most common ones below.

- **Causes of acquired spinal stenosis**

  Acquired spinal stenosis is the most common form of this condition. It tends to occur due to "wear and tear" changes that naturally occur in the spine during the aging process, especially as you navigate your 50s and 60s.

  However, other possible causes include traumatic injury, degenerative changes such as disk herniation, and iatrogenic damage (i.e. damage caused by treatments such as surgeries - in this case, laminectomy or fusion surgery). The main causes of acquired spinal stenosis include:

  - Arthritis and osteoarthritis. These chronic disorders cause several musculoskeletal changes. They damage the "cushioning" disc of cartilage that keeps the joints lubricated, thus exposing bones to friction and shock damage.

    This can lead to changes in the mechanics of the joints and lead to complications such as bone spurs. Bone spurs are an overgrowth of bone produced by the body in an attempt to repair the damage caused by cartilage loss. These bone spurs, coupled with the damage to the vertebrae caused by arthritis, can cause an abnormal, persistent narrowing of the spinal canal.

  - Bulging or herniated intervertebral discs. The intervertebral discs are flat, round cushioning pads located between the vertebrae. Their role is to absorb shock and protect the spinal bones from damage. As you age, these discs can become weaker and begin to protrude out of the spinal column. This causes bulges that press on nearby spinal nerve roots and leakages of the soft gel-like core of the intervertebral discs into the space of the spinal canal.

  - Thickened ligaments. Ligaments are strong bands of connective tissue that link one bone to another. The ligaments in the spine play a vital role in maintaining the spinal column's flexibility and resilience, while also controlling movements. Degenerative and inflammatory diseases like arthritis can have a negative effect on these ligaments, causing them to thicken, swell, and become inflamed. This can cause them to obstruct the spinal canal and limit the movement of the spine.

  - Traumatic injuries. Collisions, falls, and direct blows to the spine - which can lead to fractures and dislocations - can permanently alter the spinal structure and narrow the canal space.

- Tumors and cysts. The abnormal growth of tissue, if it occurs in and around the components of the spine, can lead to an abnormal narrowing of the canal that houses the spinal cord.

- **Causes of acquired Congenital stenosis**

  Congenital stenosis is a rarer form of this disease, reported in only 9% of cases of spinal stenosis. (15) It occurs in babies and children, and it can derive from spinal malformations that occur during fetal development and inherited conditions that affect bone growth. Some of these conditions, which are often caused by genetic modifications, include:

  - Achondroplasia. Achondroplasia is a genetic condition that results in dwarfism.
  - Spinal dysraphism. Spinal dysraphism is a broad term for a variety of developmental disorders, like spina bifida, that result from a malformation of the neural tube.
  - Congenital kyphosis. A spinal condition present at birth, characterized by an abnormal forward curvature of the spine, often resulting in a hunched or "humpback" appearance.
  - Congenital short pedicles. A rare genetic disorder in which the pedicles (the connectors of the spinal bones) are shorter than normal, potentially leading to spinal compression or instability.
  - Osteopetrosis. Also known as marble bone disease, is a rare disorder characterized by overly dense and enlarged bones.

  It is also possible to develop congenital spinal stenosis if you are born with a narrow spinal canal or if you have an abnormal curvature of the spine, which can alter spinal mechanics (scoliosis).

## Risk Factors for Spinal Stenosis

Above, I've highlighted the main causes of congenital and degenerative spinal stenosis. However, there are also some risk factors - or probable contributors - that may increase your likelihood of developing this condition. Some of these key risk factors include:

- **Aging.** As you now know, the risk of spinal stenosis increases as you get older due to the natural wear and tear of the spine that occurs over time.

- **Genetics and medical history.** If spinal stenosis runs in your family, you're more likely to develop the condition. This is also due to genetic and inheritable factors that may be passed down through generations.

- **Spine surgery.** Surgical procedures may sometimes lead to changes in spinal anatomy and scar tissue formation, which can contribute to the narrowing of the spinal canal. Spine surgery can also cause iatrogenic damage to one or more aspects of the spine.

- **Spinal injuries.** Traumas like car accidents or falls can damage the spine and increase your risk. Serious impacts can cause dislocation or fractures of one or several vertebrae. This, coupled with the ensuing swelling and inflammation, can narrow the spinal canal. You may also run the risk of developing spinal stenosis in the future if old spine injuries have not been treated properly.

- **Occupation.** Jobs that require heavy lifting or repetitive motion can stress your spine. Undue stress and overuse can speed up the degeneration of components such as the intervertebral discs, ligaments, and tendons.

- **Certain diseases.** Conditions like Paget's disease, osteoarthritis, or rheumatoid arthritis can contribute to spinal stenosis. These damage the vertebrae's joints and lead to malformations of the spine.

- **Obesity.** If you're overweight or obese, the excess weight can put extra pressure on your spine and lead to disc degeneration, as well as other changes contributing to spinal stenosis. Studies have seen a direct correlation between obesity and spinal stenosis. (6)

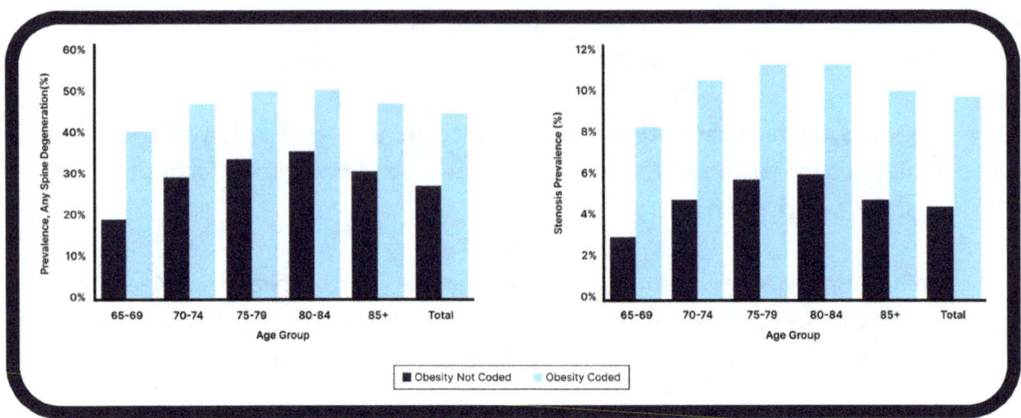


*Direct correlation between obesity and spinal stenosis*

*Data from: https://www.ncbi.nlm.nih.gov/pmc/articles/PMC7940625/*

- **Sedentary lifestyle.** Prolonged sitting and lack of exercise can weaken the muscles supporting the spine, reducing its durability. As you'll see in the prevention and treatment sections, regular physical movement helps maintain the flexibility and strength of the spine, thus mitigating the risk of spinal stenosis.

- **Smoking.** Although the relationship isn't completely understood, smoking is often associated with an increased risk of developing spinal stenosis. Smoking is also considered to be a risk factor for several degenerative conditions of the spine, and it increases all-cause mortality. (16)

- **Poor posture.** Habitual hunching or slouching modifies the mechanics of the spine and causes loads to be distributed unevenly across the spine. This can lead to conditions like bulging and herniated discs, which can narrow the spinal canal.

**Chapter 3 - Takeaways**

- Spinal stenosis is a chronic, degenerative condition of the spine that can lead to long-lasting complications, including reduced mobility, nerve damage, and disability.
- Spinal stenosis refers to an abnormal narrowing of the spinal canal, which is the passageway that houses critical nerve roots and the spinal cord itself. When these nerves are irritated or compressed, they can malfunction and lead to pain and weakness. If the entire spinal cord is compressed, patients can suffer from myelopathy, which is a serious nerve dysfunction that leads to complications like loss of bowel and bladder control.
- It mostly affects adults aged 50 and over, but anyone may be vulnerable to this condition, especially those who perform certain high-impact activities or work in specific labor-intense professions.
- Spinal stenosis is often a consequence of other degenerative conditions of the spine like intervertebral disc disease and osteoarthritis. However, spinal stenosis may also develop in its acute form if it develops due to trauma or injury.
- Spinal stenosis can also be congenital in the case of infants born with malformations of the spine or genetic mutations that affect the growth of bones.
- Risk factors for spinal stenosis include obesity, smoking, a sedentary lifestyle, poor posture, new and old trauma, and certain diseases.
- Besides the physical symptoms of spinal stenosis, patients with this condition also experience a higher risk of mental health disorders (e.g. depression), higher healthcare costs, and reduced quality of life.

# Chapter 4 - The Condition of Spinal Stenosis

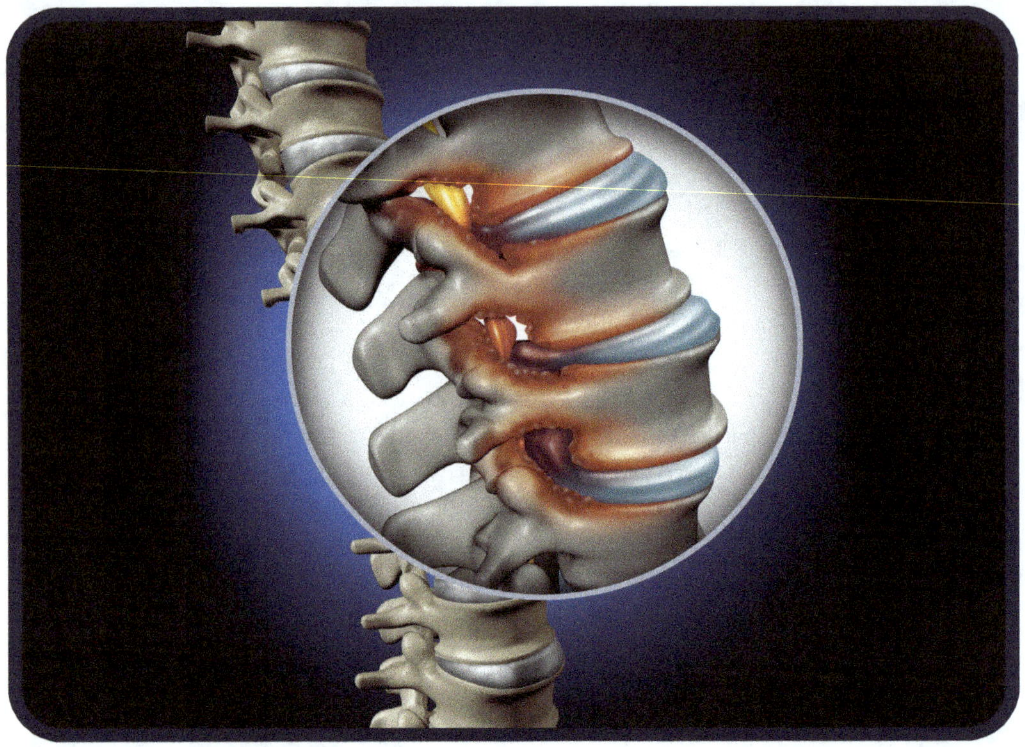

Above, I have explored the causes of spinal stenosis, and I've explained the differences between acute and chronic pain. Now, it is important to focus on the fact that the two forms of this disease - chronic spinal stenosis and acute spinal stenosis - require different approaches, have unique risk factors, and may lead to specific consequences.

Put simply, acute spinal stenosis is marked by abrupt onset, usually caused by trauma or injury. The immediate nature of this form can be alarming and often prompts swift medical attention. In severe cases, such as if the entire spinal cord is compressed, it may cause sudden paralysis or extreme pain.

On the other hand, chronic spinal stenosis is characterized by a slow development over time. The symptoms may worsen due to gradual wear and tear over months or even years. You might initially experience mild discomfort, but over time, this symptom can evolve into significant pain and mobility issues. Since chronic spinal stenosis is a slow-burning disease, it often goes unaddressed, which is the main reason why complications emerge.

Understanding the difference between acute and chronic forms of spinal stenosis is crucial. Not only does it impact how you experience and manage symptoms, but it also influences the course of treatment that doctors will recommend. Below, before looking at the treatment options available to you, I'll explain the different forms of spinal stenosis in more detail.

# Chronic Spinal Stenosis

A chronic form of spinal stenosis occurs when the narrowing of the spinal canal is caused by progressive changes in the spine. Over time, this creates immense pressure on the spinal nerves, leading to a multitude of debilitating symptoms.

To be classified as chronic, the pain you experience should last three months or longer. Spinal stenosis is considered to be one of the main causes of chronic back pain, (17) a condition that affects a quarter of the world's population and is widely considered a leading cause of disability.

| Type of LSS | Relative (≤ 12 mm) (N=191) | | Absolute (≤ 10 mm) (N=191) | |
|---|---|---|---|---|
| | N | % (95% CI) | N | % (95% CI) |
| Congenital | 9 | 4.71% (2.18-8.76%) | 5 | 2.62% (0.86-6.00%) |
| Acquired | 14 | 22.50% (16.80-29.10%) | 14 | 7.30% (4.07-11.99%) |
| Any Type | 45 | 23.60 (17.73-30.23%) | 16 | 8.40% (4.86-13.25%) |

*Selected differential diagnosis for chronic low back pain*

*Data from: https://www.aafp.org/pubs/afp/issues/2015/0515/p708.html*

One important difference between chronic and acute spinal stenosis revolves around how quickly symptoms develop. An acute case will manifest sudden, severe symptoms, often due to an injury or severe degeneration. In contrast, the symptoms of chronic spinal stenosis creep up slowly, over months, or even years.

Such slow progression often results in mild back pain and stiffness, often accompanied by numbness or weakness in the legs or arms. Recognizing these symptoms can be tricky as they're often dismissed as age-related aches and pains. The most common causes of chronic spinal stenosis certainly include disc degeneration disease and changes that occur in the spine over time.

However, several psychological and lifestyle factors may also play a role in the emergence of chronic pain conditions. For example, if you suffer from anxiety or depression, you may be more likely to develop chronic back pain or experience more intense painful sensations. (18)

If these symptoms go unnoticed, they can continue to develop, which leaves the door open to the worsening of symptoms, complications, and, eventually, severe or permanent nerve damage. When this happens, the consequences can range from physical disability to severe and constant pain, and even loss of bladder or bowel control.

What's more, suffering from chronic pain and managing your symptoms with medications can cause you to experience the side effects of medications. These side effects can be limited to tiredness and fatigue, but, in the case of NSAIDs and opioids, they can involve an increased risk of heart attack or stroke, kidney dysfunction, stomach ulcers, overdose, addiction, and death.

If you have noticed that your pain isn't improving, it is important to seek an adequate diagnosis and look for an effective treatment option that tackles the root cause of chronic pain, not just your symptoms.

# Acute Spinal Stenosis

While spinal stenosis is frequently considered to be a chronic condition, it can also develop in its acute form when its onset is sudden and rapid, usually due to a tangible health event.

Unlike chronic spinal stenosis, which develops over time due to a combination of factors, the causes of acute spinal stenosis are often easy to determine and linked to immediate trauma or injury.

For example, a car accident or a significant fall can result in a sudden change in the mechanics and structure of the spine. Studies have shown that spinal stenosis is reported in nearly 8% of car collision cases, making it one of the most common spinal injuries caused by road accidents. (19) In these cases, the cervical vertebrae are the most affected, leading to cervical spinal stenosis.

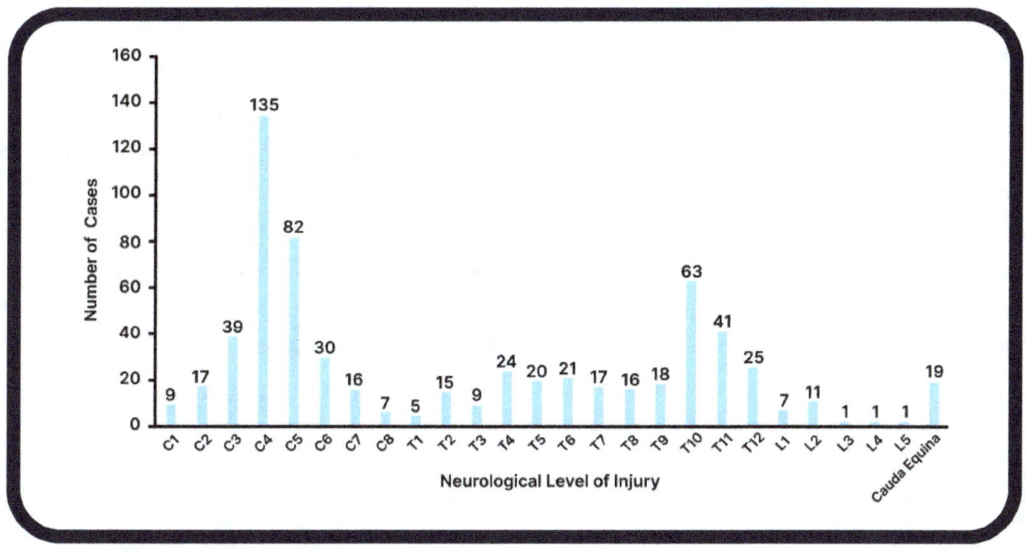


*The neurological level of motor vehicle collisions-induced spinal cord injuries, where the most common cervical spinal cord injury involved cervical 4 and cervical 5.*

*Data from: https://www.nature.com/articles/s41598-022-16930-9*

Severe injuries, even if non-traumatic or non-contact (e.g. sports injuries), can cause a quick and unexpected narrowing of the spinal canal, leading to acute spinal stenosis. In most cases, however, the pain deriving from the compression of nerves in the spinal canal or the irritation of nerve roots can be resolved by tackling the underlying traumatic injury with adequate treatment.

For example, if the narrowing of the spinal canal is due to the inflammation that ensued following a bone fracture or wound, a spacious passageway for the spinal nerves will be restored once the fracture or cut has healed.

For this, it is important to emphasize the fact that injuries require appropriate treatment to prevent long-lasting consequences. If not handled properly, these injuries could lead to long-lasting changes in the spinal canal and, in turn, chronic spinal stenosis.

Both repeated minor trauma, such as from certain sports, or major trauma can affect the spine mechanics. These altered mechanics may expedite the spine's degeneration and solidify the acute spinal stenosis into chronic pain.

In worse scenarios, untreated or improperly managed trauma can lead to permanent narrowing of the spinal canal. This can place undue pressure on nearby nerves, irritate them, and, ultimately, damage them.

Irreversible nerve damage can lead to weakness in the limbs, reduced function, and even coordination and balance problems. Tackling this problem before it develops further can help you restore the health of your spine and prevent further complications.

**Chapter 4 - Takeaways**

- Spinal stenosis can be either acute or chronic.
- Chronic spinal stenosis develops over time. It only causes mild discomfort at first, but it can progress into causing disability if not addressed. It tends to worsen alongside the condition causing it (e.g. osteoarthritis).
- Chronic spinal stenosis is a leading cause of back pain among older adults, and it's associated with a decline in mental health and quality of life.
- Some of the most common degenerative conditions at the root of spinal stenosis include osteoporosis (fractures), osteoarthritis, spondylitis, and sacroiliac joint dysfunction.
- Acute spinal stenosis is commonly a consequence of trauma or injury, such as a sports injury or car accident.
- The pain deriving from acute spinal stenosis subsides once the underlying injury is adequately addressed.
- If left unaddressed or inadequately treated, acute spinal stenosis can transform into a chronic, long-lasting condition of the spine.

# Chapter 5 - Intervention and Treatment

Spinal stenosis is a challenging condition to prevent. This is because it often emerges as a consequence of highly widespread disorders, such as arthritis or osteoarthritis. What's more, an abnormal narrowing of the spinal canal isn't always adequately diagnosed before prescribing treatment for chronic or acute back pain.

Because of this, it isn't always easy to identify the strategies that would help you keep your spine safe. Nonetheless, there are certain approaches that are proven to be beneficial in maintaining overall spine health, flexibility, and durability. These approaches can help you boost your musculoskeletal well-being, reduce your functional disability, and prevent chronic pain conditions.

In the following sections, I'll look at the goal of preventive measures for spinal stenosis as well as ad hoc strategies that you can put into practice today to prevent the most impactful consequences of this condition.

## Preventative Measures

Spinal stenosis cannot always be easily prevented. Nonetheless, the prevention of degenerative spine disease is considered to be the most powerful tool to reduce the complications of the narrowing of the spinal canal, prevent disability, and ease the burden of low back pain conditions on the national healthcare system.

Preventive measures for spinal stenosis don't only have the goal of avoiding the emergence of the disease. Additional goals could be to:

- **Prevent injury and reinjury of the spine.** This aspect is particularly prominent among patients who are at risk of trauma and injuries that may lead to acute spinal stenosis. The demographics at risk may be workers who put their spines under frequent excessive mechanical load, athletes, and older adults.

- **Prevent complications and comorbidities.** Adequate management of spinal stenosis can prevent some of its most severe complications, such as nerve damage or disability. What's more, by implementing certain preventive measures, patients can reduce the risk of comorbidities commonly seen with spinal stenosis, including certain forms of arthritis and joint damage.

- **Support spine health.** Most of the prevention strategies available focus on implementing positive changes that support the overall health of the spine and of the musculoskeletal system as a whole. For example, adequate posture, regular exercise, weight management, and mental health check-ups can do a lot to reduce the risk of chronic musculoskeletal conditions.

## Preventative Measures for Chronic Spinal Stenosis

As I explained above, spinal stenosis can derive from chronic conditions of the spine such as osteoarthritis and arthritis. Given that the majority of people show signs of spine osteoarthritis by the age of 50, it can be extremely difficult to prevent a chronic form of spinal stenosis from developing.

Nonetheless, there are some simple strategies that can be introduced to reduce the risk of spinal disease and increase the number of years lived without disability.

These strategies are:

- **Make exercise a part of your daily routine.**

If dealing with spinal stenosis, incorporating exercise into your everyday schedule is an essential step. Not only does physical activity enhance your general health, help you keep a healthy weight, and reduce the risk of diseases like diabetes and obesity - but it also specifically fortifies your spine too.

Regular exercise increases your core strength and boosts flexibility, reducing the risk of developing spinal stenosis and other spine-related conditions.
What's more, exercises directed at alleviating spinal stenosis may help you better withstand mechanical loads, improve posture, reduce pain-related disability, and foster stronger, more elastic muscles. Ideally, you'll want to practice both aerobic, low-impact exercises and strength training.

The foundations of an exercise program for spinal stenosis should include:

- Hamstring stretches. These ease tight lower back muscles and reduce pressure on your lumbar spine.
- Lumbar flexion and lengthening. Known as "backward bending," this exercise decompresses spinal nerves.
- Core strengthening. Core strengthening exercises like crunches and planks can help you engage your core and strengthen the muscles of your upper and central body. This is important to provide the spine with the necessary support.
- Pilates or yoga. These mind-body disciplines can help you strengthen and lengthen the muscles of your body, but they can also help you boost coordination, balance, and proprioception, which are essential aspects to help you reduce the risk of falls and injuries.
- Aerobic exercises. Low-impact activities like swimming or cycling can provide cardiovascular benefits without straining your spine.
- Stretching. Stretching is a powerful tool to boost the flexibility and resilience of your spine. Stretching exercises can help you reduce the risk of falls and other forms of injuries, but they can also help you reduce disability and boost the function of the spine.

Last but not least, stretching and massaging your tense muscles may help relieve the pressure on the nerves in and around the spinal area, which can relieve the symptoms of back pain and discomfort.

If any of the options above seem difficult or undesirable to you, you may consider finding an activity you truly enjoy - after all, the goal is to keep moving!

- **Focus on maintaining good posture**

Good posture plays a pivotal role in maintaining the health of your spine. When you sit or stand with correct alignment, you minimize strain on your spinal structures and allow mechanical loads to be distributed evenly across the spinal structure, thus avoiding undue stress on delicate components (e.g. the intervertebral discs).

Persistent poor posture can lead to spinal stenosis, among other spine-related conditions, by increasing stress on your spinal column.

Because of this, several of the prevention strategies used to reduce the risk of spinal stenosis focus on improving posture, especially when performing sports, lifting objects, sitting, or standing.

Besides learning how to properly lift objects to avoid injuries, posture-improving exercises include:

- Shoulder blade squeezes
- Neck stretches
- Waxing
- Wall slide
- Sit to stand
- Cat cow
- Chest opener
- High plank
- Child's pose

- **Maintain a healthy weight**

As seen above, there is a direct correlation between a high body mass index (BMI) - which characterizes obesity and being overweight - and spinal stenosis, among other conditions of the spine. Because of this, keeping a healthy weight is critical for your spine health disease prevention.

Excessive weight on your torso puts immense, undue pressure on your spine, leading to issues like spinal stenosis. What's more, being obese or overweight is a risk factor for a whole host of other chronic diseases, including cardiovascular disease, osteoarthritis, and diabetes, all of which can take a toll on your musculoskeletal health.

As a preventive method to lower the risk of spinal stenosis, consider losing any excess weight and maintain a healthy BMI by:

- <u>Exercising regularly.</u> Ideally, mix aerobic exercise with strength training to burn calories and tone your body. Being more active can also reduce the risk of cardiovascular disease and boost your endurance, as well as having positive effects on your mental health.

- Switching up your diet. Implement the principles of a Mediterranean diet: focus on whole grains, fruits, vegetables, and legumes; avoid processed foods and red meats; minimize the consumption of animal products.

- Focusing on hydration, sleep, and stress management. Making sleep, stress reduction, and hydration priorities in your life can reduce inflammation and boost your levels of energy, thus making it easier to shed any excess weight you may be carrying.

If in doubt, partnering with a specialized nutritionist should always be considered the first port of call for a successful weight loss journey.

- **Quit smoking**

Cigarette smoke contains chemicals that can interfere with your body's calcium absorption, which is a crucial element for your bone health, including your spine. Also, nicotine can restrict blood flow, causing spine degeneration, slow healing of spinal injuries, and nerve damage (neurotoxicity). Studies have also highlighted a direct correlation between smoking and intervertebral disc degeneration. (20)

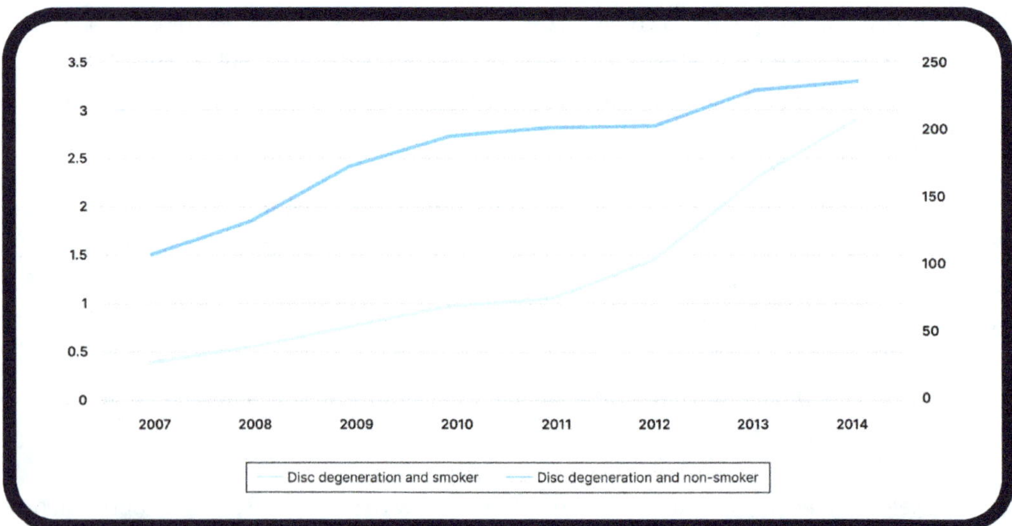


*Incidence of patients who smoke vs. non-smokers with degenerative disc disease per 10,000 patients.*

*Data from: https://www.asianspinejournal.org/journal/view.php?number=227*

If you are looking to reduce your consumption of tobacco or quit smoking, some options include using nicotine patches, finding support from a quitline, working with a mental health professional, and improving your whole environment to remove triggers.

### Preventative Measures for Acute Spinal Stenosis

Some of the preventive measures seen above - those that aim to boost overall spine health - are applicable to acute spinal stenosis too. However, in addition to quitting smoking and shedding extra weight, there are also some specific preventive measures that can help you reduce the risk of suffering from acute spinal stenosis.

These measures, which focus on reducing the likelihood of falls, accidents, and traumatic injuries involving the spine, include:

- **Assessing occupational risks.** Studies have shown that certain occupations, such as machine drivers and carpenters, have a higher risk of degenerative conditions of the spine, including disc degeneration and spinal stenosis. (21)

  You can mitigate this risk by carrying out a thorough risk assessment at work to identify potential hazards (e.g. lifting heavy objects) and using the necessary personal protective equipment. You may also introduce exercise programs and training courses that may help reduce the burden of low back pain in your workspace.

- **Improving your athletic form.** Certain sports require athletes to perform sudden and forceful movements that place excessive stress on the spine, thus accelerating the degeneration of components such as the intervertebral discs.

  These sports include football, basketball, and soccer, but cases of cervical spinal stenosis have also been found among professional rugby league players, as a consequence of traumatic injuries. (22)

  To reduce the level of risk, consider improving your form, partnering with a specialist to boost your physical form, and wearing the necessary protective equipment. If you are struggling with spine problems and chronic pain, you may also need to consider solutions such as activity modifications to limit the strain on your spine.

- **Improving strength, balance, coordination, and flexibility.** Especially among elderly patients, a leading cause of acute spinal stenosis is falls and slips that cause spine damage.

  For example, among older people, fractures of the pelvis and hip are extremely common injuries that occur as a consequence of falls. To reduce the risk of falls it is important to improve mobility and, to do so, patients should follow comprehensive exercise programs that include balance, coordination, flexibility, and strength exercises.

  Disciplines such as yoga and tai chi may be great starting options for elderly patients looking to become more active. The use of home safety features (such as rails and mobility-friendly bathtubs) may also reduce the risk of household injuries.

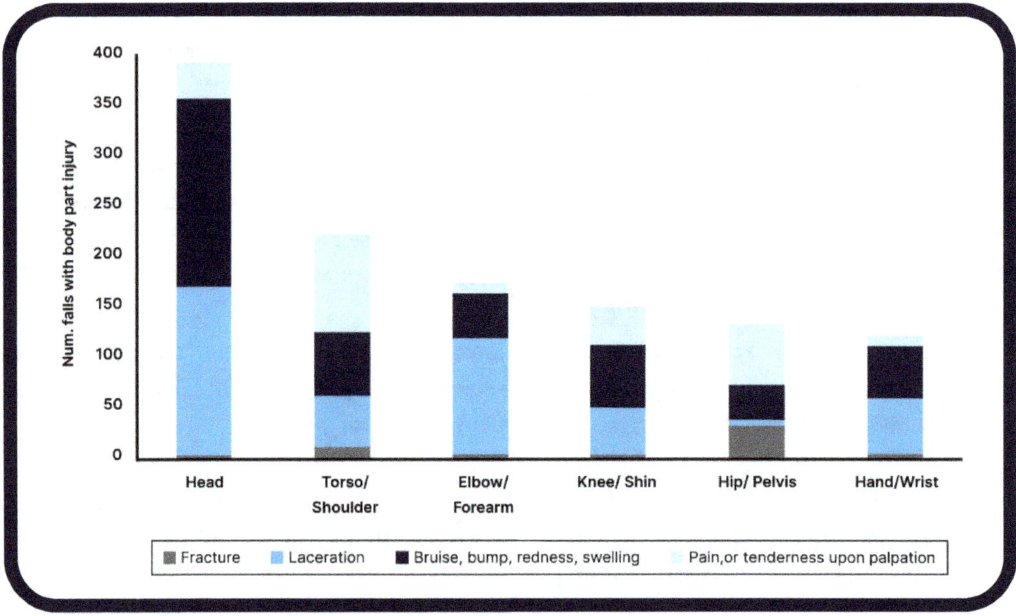


*Injury distribution by body part and injury type.*

*Data from: https://bmcgeriatr.biomedcentral.com/articles/10.1186/s12877-022-03041-3*

**Chapter 5 - Takeaways**

- Preventive measures play a vital role in reducing the risk of degenerative back disease and promoting overall spine health.
- Since most adults will develop osteoarthritis as they age, it is not possible to totally prevent degenerative conditions of the spine, such as spinal stenosis.
- Some preventive measures for chronic spinal stenosis include maintaining a healthy weight, making exercise part of your routine, practicing strength and flexibility training for the spine, maintaining a good posture, and quitting smoking.
- Preventive measures for acute spinal stenosis focus on reducing the risk of injuries and household accidents. These include practicing strength and flexibility training, improving athletic form, and assessing any occupational risks.

# Chapter 6 - Conventional Treatment Options

Today, most patients with spinal stenosis face a significant delay in obtaining an adequate diagnosis of their disease. And when the diagnosis comes, often, healthcare providers suggest managing the symptoms through pain medications and inefficient therapies. This choice can lead to a cascade of side effects.

Firstly, medications come with severe side effects, which can lead to even more worrisome conditions and health complications. Additionally, not tackling the root of the problem means that most patients have a single prospect ahead of them: living with chronic pain and hoping to never require surgery.

Unfortunately, for many, this isn't the case: on average, 37% to 52% of patients with spinal stenosis require surgery to recover some of their spine function and reduce pain. (23)

Nonetheless, there are options to reduce the need for surgery and find adequate treatment that truly tackles the root cause of spinal degeneration. It all starts with **recognizing spinal stenosis as a severe condition that requires immediate care.**

This approach will help you prevent an acute injury from transforming into a persistent chronic disorder and lead to health complications. In the sections below, I'll explore some of the most commonly prescribed treatment plans for spinal stenosis, and I'll highlight their efficiency and limitations.

## Non-Surgical vs Surgical Treatment Options

Spinal stenosis can be treated either surgically or non-surgically. The choice of approach will depend on the severity of your condition and pain, as well as whether your discomfort is causing your disability or mobility issues.

Additionally, you may require surgery if you have been diagnosed with some of the complications of spinal stenosis, such as radiculopathy or spondylosis (neck pain caused by the abnormal wear and tear of the cartilage in the vertebrae of the neck).

Here's how the two options compare.

## Non-Surgical Management of Spinal Stenosis

Non-surgical management of spinal stenosis has a main goal: relieving painful symptoms by temporarily reducing the levels of inflammation and swelling. These medications can help you better manage your symptoms during painful flare-ups or while waiting for a better treatment approach.

Non-surgical therapies may be recommended in the event of mild spinal stenosis, when the nerve roots are only minimally affected and the pain is bearable. If the entire spinal cord is compressed or you are experiencing disabling pain and mobility problems, you may be recommended to undergo surgery.

## Surgical Management of Spinal Stenosis

There are several surgical options to manage spinal stenosis, including laminectomy and spinal decompression, surgeries that aim to free up or relieve the pressure on affected nerves. These are usually recommended when the pain is causing disability or getting in the way of a patient's life.

However, it is important to keep in mind that no surgical intervention is entirely free of risk - nor can clinical outcomes be exactly foreseen.

| Case No. | Sex | Age (y) | Decompressed Level | Comorbidity |
|---|---|---|---|---|
| 1 | F | 38 | L5-S1 | Diabetes |
| 2 | F | 60 | L3-L5 | Hypertension, coronary artery disease |
| 3 | M | 75 | L4-S1 | Hypertension |
| 4 | F | 84 | L2-L5 | Antiphospholipid, hypertension, coronary artery disease |
| 5 | F | 49 | L4-L5 | Fatty liver |

***Demographics of patients with postoperative cauda equina syndrome***

*Data from: https://www.ncbi.nlm.nih.gov/pmc/articles/PMC3864468/*



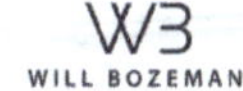

For example, studies have shown that cauda equina syndrome is a complication in nearly 3% of spinal decompression surgeries for spinal stenosis. (24) Cauda equina is a serious neurological condition caused by the compression of nerve roots in the lower spine.

A medical emergency, this condition can cause potential long-term effects, including loss of bladder and bowel control, sexual dysfunction, and even paralysis if left untreated.

Additionally, all surgical interventions involving the spine will come with lengthy recovery and rehabilitation periods.

# NSAIDs

If you're suffering from spinal stenosis, NSAIDs are likely to play a large role in your treatment plan. Nonsteroidal anti-inflammatory drugs (NSAIDs) are a type of medication capable of temporarily reducing inflammation and relieving pain.

NSAIDs work by blocking certain body enzymes known as COX-1 and COX-2. By causing the production of prostaglandins - chemicals that mediate inflammation - these enzymes contribute to inflammation and pain in the body. When these enzymes are inhibited, you'll experience a significant reduction in discomfort.

### Efficacy and Safety

By taking NSAIDs, you can enjoy increased mobility and a decrease in the pain caused by spinal stenosis. Remember, though, that while NSAIDs can be highly beneficial, they're not a cure-all. They are a supportive measure that only provides symptomatic relief.

Not only are NSAIDs affordable and easily available as over-the-counter alternatives, but they can also be a valid pain management option when you are experiencing back pain flare-ups or just after an injury.

However, it's important to keep in mind that these medications don't modify or cure the disease, and, when taken in the long term, they can lead to significant risks and side effects. These include an increased risk of heart attack and stroke, kidney dysfunction, heart failure, stomach ulcers, and addiction. (25)

# Corticosteroid Injections

Simply, corticosteroid injections work by decreasing inflammation and, in turn, pain and swelling. Corticosteroids are the manufactured version of cortisol, a hormone that is naturally found in the body. This hormone is responsible for medicating inflammation and pain, as well as playing a role in the immune system response.

Corticosteroid injections are usually delivered into the painful joint using imaging guidance methods like X-rays. They work by decreasing the immune response in the affected area, thus temporarily reducing inflammation. The injection is composed of slow-release chemicals that will deliver anti-inflammatory steroids over time, thus leading to a longer-lasting effect compared to standard pain medications.

### Efficacy and Safety

Corticosteroid injections may seem like a great pain management option, especially if you are waiting for spinal surgery or you are experimenting with different treatment options. Nonetheless, these injections should never be considered a long-term solution for degenerative conditions of the spine.

Not only do steroids do very little to modify the underlying disease, but they come with severe side effects. These include:

- **Adrenal insufficiency.** This is a serious condition that occurs when the adrenal glands, which are the glands in charge of producing cortisol, don't work as they should. (26)
- **Progression of joint diseases.** Injections of corticosteroids into the joint can speed up the progression of joint diseases like osteoarthritis. In turn, these can aggravate spinal stenosis and other degenerative diseases of the spine.
- **Inhibited stem cells.** Corticosteroids can have an inhibiting effect on stem cells. (27) This inhibiting effect interferes with your body's natural healing mechanisms, increases inflammation, and slows healing rates. If you are considering stem cell treatments, steroid injections might even counteract this therapy.

# Opioids

Opioids are a type of medication that contains an active ingredient naturally found in the opium poppy plant. They work by attaching to special receptors in your brain, spinal cord, and other areas of your body. This connection interferes with the perception of pain, offering some relief to those suffering from spinal stenosis. By limiting the ability of your nervous system to communicate pain, you feel less discomfort.

If you are struggling with chronic pain, there is a high chance that your doctor will, at some point, prescribe opioids to help you cope with the discomfort and mobility problems.

As shown in the graph below, the number of patients taking opioids for degenerative back disorders declines in the months after diagnosis, and it can even be further reduced by undergoing surgery.

Nonetheless, today, as many as two-thirds of patients with non-specific low back or neck pain receive an opioid when presenting for care. (28) More specifically, the number of opioid-based analgesics for lumbar spinal stenosis has been on the rise since 2018. (29)

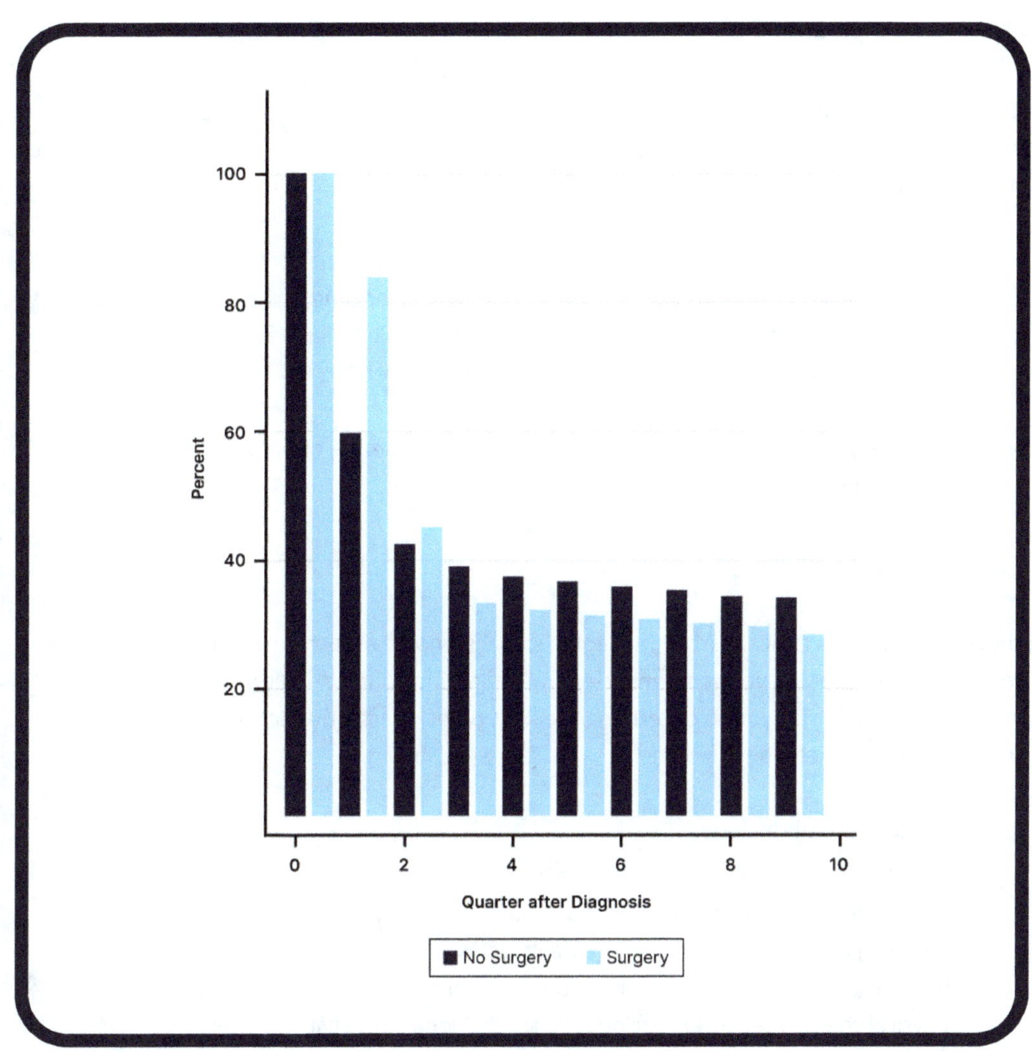


*A histogram illustrating the use of opioids, where the proportion of patients who had used opioids declined with time after the diagnosis date.*

*Data from: https://link.springer.com/article/10.1007/s00586-023-07901-3*

### Efficacy and Safety

In the case of flare-ups - and when highly regulated by a physician - this class of drugs may help you regain spine mobility. However, given the severe side effects they can cause, as well as the fact that these medications don't modify the disease, opioids should not be considered as the ultimate solution for spinal stenosis.

Some side effects of opioids include nausea, vomiting, and constipation. More critically, long-term use can lead to physical dependence and addiction. Over time, the body can develop tolerance, requiring higher doses to experience the same pain relief effect. This can lead to dependence and in worst-case scenarios, an overdose or death.

Because of this, proper regulation is crucial for safety. Your usage of opioids for managing spinal stenosis should always be monitored by a physician.

## Physical Therapy

Physical therapy is a critical part of managing spinal stenosis, as it focuses on boosting spine health by strengthening your core muscles and improving your flexibility. Your physical therapist will work with you to determine the best types of activities and exercises for your unique musculoskeletal needs.

However, these usually include:

- Stretching exercises to improve your flexibility
- Aerobic exercises to increase your overall endurance
- Strength training to bolster your core muscles
- Posture correction to reduce strain on your spine
- Physical therapy-led interventions like tai-chi, yoga, and Pilates
- Athletic form correction
- Occupational therapy to reduce exposure to risks in the workplace

Physical therapy can significantly aid in improving your body's endurance and flexibility. This helps reduce the strain on your spine, which can prevent the condition from worsening. The various exercises may also relieve pressure on the nerves and the spinal cord, thus immediately offering relief from pain.

### Efficacy and Safety

Physical therapy, when carried out by a specialized physician, can be extremely beneficial to support overall spine health.

When coupled with other interventions like yoga or tai-chi, physical therapy can help patients strengthen their muscles and boost their flexibility, and it may even boost balance, coordination, symmetry, and proprioception (the awareness of the position of the body within the surrounding space).

These positive effects can reduce the risk of falls, which can injure or re-injure the spine.

The only drawbacks of physical therapy you should keep in mind are temporary muscle soreness, minor dehydration, and fatigue after a session, as well as the risk of injury when treatment is performed by an unqualified professional.

## Icing and Heat

Ice and heat are common at-home remedies for back or neck pain, including the type of discomfort caused by spinal stenosis. Although these methods may not help cure your condition, they are considered relatively safe ways to ease your symptoms without medications, especially during flare-ups.

Heat therapy can soothe stiff spinal muscles and joints, thus relieving nerve strain and irritation. Heat compresses work by increasing blood flow to the affected area, which consequently accelerates healing by delivering more nutrients to the affected area. Additionally, heat can improve flexibility and decrease muscle spasms and tightness.

Ice therapy can also prove extremely useful. Unlike heat which promotes blood flow, ice significantly reduces it. This in turn results in lowered swelling and inflammation in the area where you experience pain. What's more, reduced swelling can free up space in the spinal canal, thus providing immediate relief from discomfort.



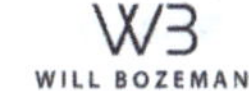

When it comes to applying these treatments at home, start with placing hot or cold compresses on the part of the spine affected by pain for around 10-20 minutes each time. You can repeat this treatment multiple times a day, but be sure to listen to your body and follow the instructions of your healthcare provider. If you notice worsening pain, discomfort, or skin irritation, immediately interrupt the treatment and call your doctor.

### Efficacy and Safety

While both heat and ice therapy bring relief to spinal stenosis, these methods are not devoid of potential risks or limitations. Overuse of heat can cause burns or blistering, while extremely cold compresses might lead to skin damage or frostbite. Moreover, these treatments may not be ideal for everyone, particularly for those with pre-existing skin conditions or poor circulatory health.

## Laminectomy

Laminectomy is a common surgical procedure used to alleviate the pain and discomfort associated with spinal stenosis. This operation aims to create more space for the nerves of the spinal cord by removing a portion of the vertebrae forming the spinal canal. The procedure involves making a small incision in the back, after which the surgeon carefully removes the bony arches of your vertebrae.

After the surgery, the spinal cord and nerves have more space, which can reduce the pressure on the nerve roots and restore their function, partially or entirely. In turn, this can significantly reduce symptoms like pain, numbness, and muscle weakness. Recovery from a laminectomy usually takes a few weeks, and you may be required to follow physical therapy or specific exercises to strengthen your back.

### Efficacy and Safety

Laminectomy is one of the most popular types of surgery performed for spinal stenosis. This invasive intervention has the ultimate goal of improving your quality of life, and, in general, most people are able to experience significant relief from their symptoms and return to their daily activities.

Nonetheless, like all forms of surgery, you'll run the risk of infections, negative reactions to the anesthetic drugs used during the surgery, and complications such as nerve damage. It is also important to keep in mind two aspects of laminectomy:

- The efficacy of laminectomy - whether or not it is combined with spinal fusion - largely depends on how severe your case of spinal stenosis was before surgery and whether you are also suffering from complications like cervical spondylotic myelopathy. (30)
- Low back (lumbar) laminectomy, when performed without spinal fusion, can lead to the risk of adjacent segment disease (ASD), which is prevalent in up to 10% of patients undergoing this type of surgery. (31) ASD is a potential complication of spinal surgery. It occurs when the segments of your spine adjacent to the surgery site start to break down. This causes discomfort and similar symptoms to those that led to surgery in the first place, thus requiring revision surgery.

# Laminotomy

Laminotomy is a surgical method that revolves around removing a portion of the lamina, which is the back part of your vertebra that covers your spinal canal.

During the procedure, a small cut is made in the skin of the back to provide access to the affected vertebra. The surgeon then delicately removes either part or all of the lamina. This creates more room in the spinal canal, thus relieving pressure on irritated or compressed nerves. When successful, this surgery can lead to a significant reduction in symptoms like pain, numbness, and weakness.

### Efficacy and Safety

Laminotomy can lead to positive clinical outcomes, and it is considered successful in reducing symptoms in over 80% of the cases - a high percentage when compared to the 64% success rate of traditional laminectomy. What's more, compared to laminectomy, laminotomy (especially when performed for lumbar spinal stenosis) has been seen to lead to a lower complication rate and higher levels of patient satisfaction. (32)

Nonetheless, just like any surgical procedure, it can come with potential risks and complications like nerve damage and infections. Other possible risks include blood clots, bleeding, or anesthesia complications.

# Laminoplasty

Laminoplasty is another surgical procedure commonly used to alleviate the symptoms of spinal stenosis through spinal decompression. It works by creating space in your spinal canal by reshaping, instead of removing, the lamina. During the procedure, the lamina is cut to create a hinge or opening, which creates more space for the spinal cord to run freely. Then the surgeon will use a bone graft or metal screws to fix the opening and provide stability to the spine.

### Efficacy and Safety

Over the past years, the levels of safety and accuracy of laminoplasty have increased, and the time necessary to perform the surgery - as well as the length of hospital stay following the surgery - have decreased. This makes it an ever more valid alternative to laminectomy and laminotomy.

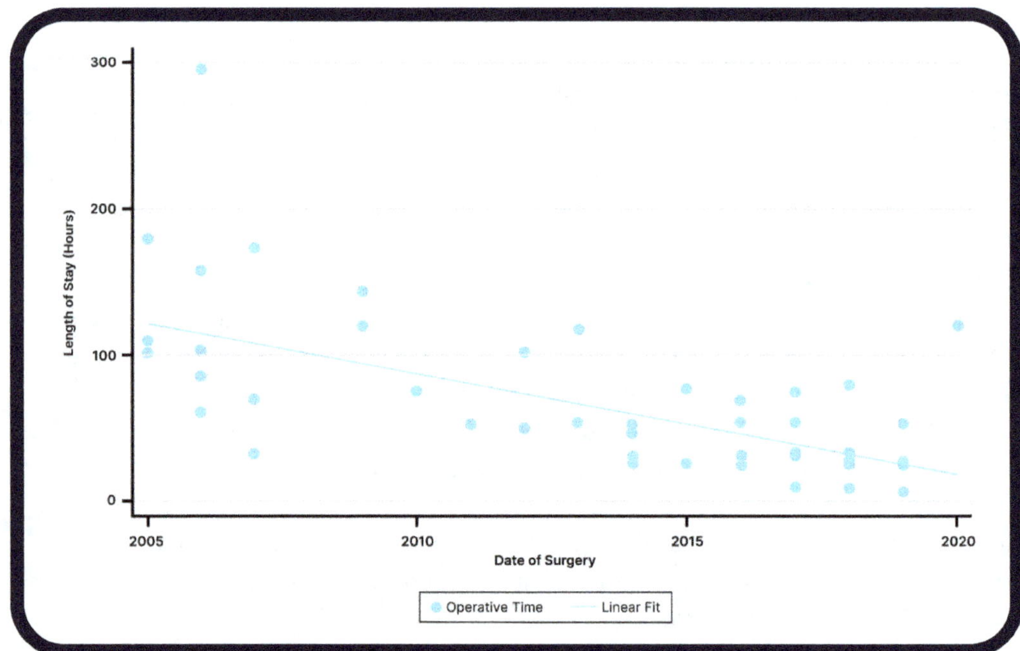


*Cervical laminoplasty operative time*

*Data from: https://journaloei.scholasticahq.com/article/17139-feasibility-of-outpatient-cervical-laminoplasty*

Nonetheless, laminoplasty is a highly invasive procedure that involves the reshaping of several vertebrae. Not only does this involve lengthy recovery times, but it also comes with risks such as permanent nerve root damage, blood clotting, reduced clinical outcomes, and infections.

**Chapter 6 - Takeaways**

- Depending on the severity of spinal stenosis and on the presence of comorbidities, you may be recommended to follow a surgical or nonsurgical treatment plan.
- Non-surgical treatments are recommended in the case of mild spinal stenosis and minor discomfort. Surgery may be needed if you are experiencing disability, severe pain, or a disorder that isn't responding to medications.
- Nonsurgical pharmacological interventions for spinal stenosis include NSAIDs, corticosteroid injections, and opioids.
- Nonsurgical, non-drug interventions include physical therapy and icing or heat.
- Surgical interventions to decompress the spine and restore space in the spinal canal include laminectomy, laminotomy, and laminoplasty.

# Chapter 7 - Unconventional Treatment Options

Besides the treatment options I've explained above, there are also some unconventional therapies that can help you better manage your symptoms while reducing the need for medications. These include massage therapy, acupuncture, and nutraceuticals as well as osteopathic and chiropractic care.

While these therapies are generally considered safe - when administered by specialists - they come with downsides worth being aware of. Aside from the fact that these therapies may not be equally efficient for all patients nor lead to the desired results, they can also carry health risks due to the limited studies and regulations in existence today.

What's more, all of the therapies highlighted in the following sections are inefficient when administered alone, without significant lifestyle modifications, exercise programs, and, in some cases, medications.

While, in most cases, it is **safe to try unconventional approaches for spinal stenosis, be sure to use them as part of a more comprehensive, multidisciplinary line of treatment.**

## Nutraceuticals

Nutraceuticals are a type of alternative medicine, which use food or food products to provide health and medical benefits. These supplements claim to have beneficial effects for certain disorders (e.g. spinal stenosis or osteoarthritis), and they are meant to enhance your health, delay the aging process, prevent chronic diseases, increase life expectancy, or even support the functioning of your body.

These supplements are taken orally, and their consumption should be closely monitored by a specialized physician to avoid allergic reactions and other adverse effects on a patient's health, such as interference with other medications. What's more, it is important to keep in mind that the efficiency of nutraceuticals is dictated by the willingness of a patient to make positive changes in their lifestyle and follow a healthy diet.

The nutraceuticals commonly recommended for degenerative back disease or spinal stenosis include supplements like vitamins B12, B9, C, and D as well as nutrients like magnesium and omega-3 fatty acids. Additionally, certain supplements - like glucosamine and chondroitin - have been historically used in the treatment of conditions like osteoarthritis which, as we have seen above, can increase the risk of spinal stenosis.

These supplements can also help reduce the risk of deficiencies that are correlated to an increased risk of spinal stenosis. In particular, studies have shown that nearly three-quarters of patients with lumbar spinal stenosis have low levels of vitamin D, a deficiency that also worsens osteoporosis, increases the likelihood of fractures, and heightens the perception of pain. (33)

### Efficacy and Safety

The safety and effectiveness of health supplements, or nutraceuticals, are still being examined. Regulatory bodies are still in the process of crafting guidelines for the safe use of nutraceuticals, while new studies often lead to controversies.

This has been the case for glucosamine sulfate and chondroitin methylsulfonylmethane, two compounds that have been commonly recommended for osteoarthritis over the past years.

New research is now highlighting the negative effects of these nutraceuticals, and, today, the Arthritis Foundation "strongly recommends against the use of glucosamine alone or in combination with chondroitin for osteoarthritis." (34)

Ultimately, the medical community keeps a skeptical eye on these products, for several reasons, including:

- Companies making flashy promises and using tactics such as celebrity backing and pyramid selling
- The limited evidence and clinical trials available to certify these companies' claims
- The emergence of new studies that prove certain health claims to be false
- The wrong beliefs of consumers that these nutraceuticals will protect them from complications or diseases, thus getting in the way of patients accessing the medical care they need

The FDA makes sure companies aren't misleading about what their products can do. But this doesn't change the fact that we - both healthcare providers and patients - need more proof before nutraceuticals can be recognized as accepted, safe treatments.

# Chiropractic Care

Chiropractic care is a form of alternative treatment that involves the physical manipulation of the body's structures, particularly the spine, to re-establish correct mechanics. It corrects the misalignments in the body's muscular and skeletal structure, which can aid in alleviating pain and discomfort.

Performed by chiropractic specialists, this type of treatment can be used to ease the symptoms of degenerative conditions of the spine, especially if they are caused by inadequate posture or changes in how loads are distributed.

### Efficacy and Safety

When performed by a qualified practitioner, chiropractic care is generally considered a safe method of treatment for many musculoskeletal issues, including spinal stenosis and other degenerative conditions of the spine. It may help patients by re-establishing the correct mechanics of the spine, which can alleviate the pressure on the nerves of the spinal cord and provide immediate relief from pain and numbness.

Nonetheless, like any other form of treatment, this approach isn't entirely free of risks. One of the main problems you may face is choosing an unqualified or inexperienced practitioner.

Besides soreness and discomfort at the adjustment site, inadequate chiropractic care can worsen the symptoms of spinal stenosis by leading to nerve damage, nerve compression, and disc herniation. If you are looking to try chiropractic care for cervical spinal stenosis, you should also be aware of the fact that neck manipulation can - in rare cases - lead to a certain type of stroke. (35)

# Osteopathic Care

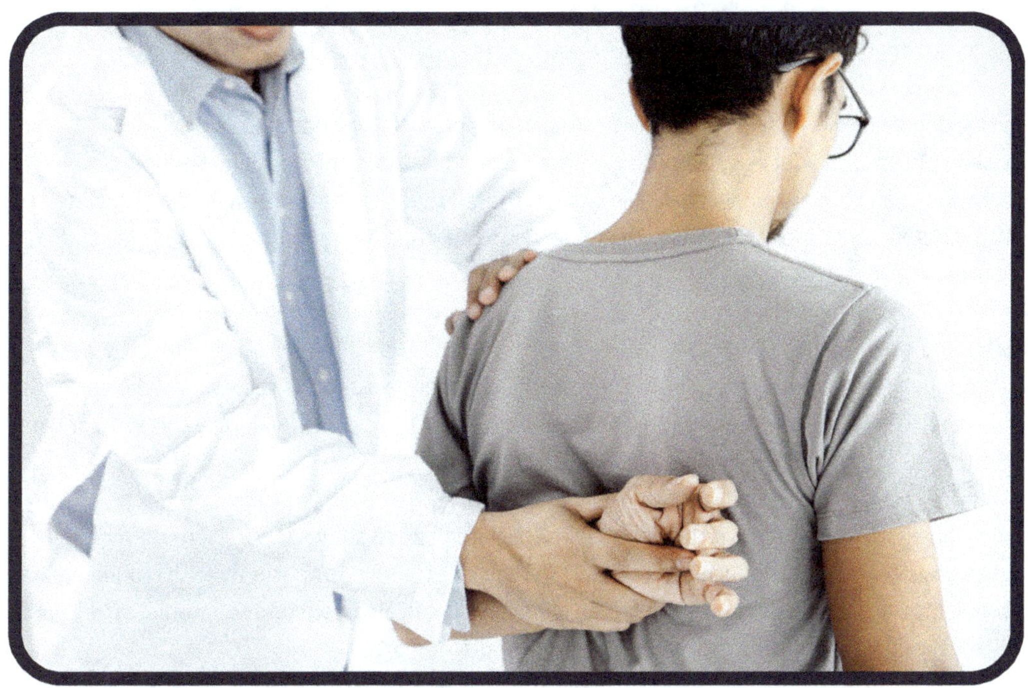

Originating from a recognized medical discipline, osteopathic care encompasses manipulative practices performed by Doctors of Osteopathic Medicine (DOs). DOs are healthcare professionals specifically trained in the techniques of manipulation, massage, and delicate stretching. Used in combination, these techniques may help in:

- Adjusting the body's mechanics and establishing balance in how the different parts of the body work together
- Boosting blood circulation, as well as the supply of nutrients and oxygen to the areas affected by pain
- Relieving muscle tension and pressure on nerves

Osteopathic care is often associated with chiropractic care, but the two forms of therapy are significantly different. Although both fields utilize manual treatment, their core approaches differ.

For instance, osteopathic care involves a comprehensive, holistic approach to wellness and prevention, targeting the interconnectedness of the musculoskeletal system's varying components - bones, muscles, ligaments, and connective tissue. On the other hand, chiropractors use manipulation to adjust your spine and joint position.

In treating spinal stenosis, osteopathic care can be beneficial. It boosts the body's self-healing potential, reduces systemic inflammation, and reduces chronic pain. Besides simply restoring space in the spinal canal, this type of therapy can also ease the swelling associated with inflammation and strengthen the spine structure, thus preventing future injuries and disorders.

### Efficacy and Safety

Although more research is required to establish whether osteopathic care is a valid treatment for spine conditions, it is undeniable that most patients choosing to integrate this type of care into their treatment plan see significant benefits.

Additionally, a systematic literature review published in 2018 shows that, although more research is needed, osteopathic manipulation may be effective for patients with spinal complaints, especially those with low back pain. (36) It can also help patients reduce their reliance on pain medications to manage pain and discomfort.

Nonetheless, it is crucial to keep in mind that osteopathic care may not be suitable for all patients. What's more, osteopathic care for spinal stenosis may also carry risks, particularly if it involves neck manipulation. This technique could lead to severe complications like nerve damage and even trigger strokes in rare cases.

## Diet and Activity Modification

Your lifestyle, sports activities, and job can greatly influence your spine health. For example, if you frequently carry heavy items or partake in high-impact sports, you'll notice that your activities will eventually take a toll on your spine health. Even something as routine as sitting at a desk all day can strain your spine over time.

Additionally, while a nutritious diet can support spine health, inadequate eating can add fuel to the fire of inflammation. Foods high in sugar and unhealthy fats can heighten inflammation in your body. This inflammation can worsen the pain and swelling in the spine, which can worsen your symptoms and further narrow your spinal canal.

Because of this, modifying your diet and lifestyle can help you ease your symptoms and regain spine function naturally and without medications. Some strategies to help you get started include:

- Practicing low-impact sports
- Focusing on anti-inflammatory foods (e.g. increasing the consumption of fresh fruits, vegetables, and legumes while reducing the intake of processed foods, alcoholic drinks, and animal products)
- Switching your tasks at work to reduce strain on the spine
- Working with a nutritionist or personal trainer

## Efficacy and Safety

Modifying your lifestyle is generally safe. However, this approach to easing the symptoms of spinal stenosis has its own set of limitations that you should keep in mind when integrating it into your treatment plan.

Firstly, not everyone can change their lifestyle significantly and promptly. For example, professional athletes whose livelihoods rely on their participation in a certain sport may not be able to switch activities overnight. The same scenario applies to certain specialists, such as carpenters or technicians who may not be able to change careers or job positions immediately.

What's more, a DIY approach to diet and activity modification can lead to drawbacks such as nutritional deficiency and higher levels of inactivity, which can have a counterproductive effect on the spine and your musculoskeletal health as a whole. If in doubt, partnering with specialists can help you prevent these risks and optimize health outcomes.

# Acupuncture and Herbal Medicine

Acupuncture and herbal medicine, two well-renowned modalities of traditional Chinese medicine (TCM), can offer significant relief for spinal stenosis. Grounded in centuries-old practices, these treatments target the patient's overall well-being, offering a holistic approach to health care.

In particular, acupuncture can ease muscle tension and relieve pressure on irritated nerves. It is performed by specialists who target pressure points that correlate to pain perception, boosting the body's natural pain relief mechanisms.

Similarly, herbal medicine offers an avenue of relief for spinal stenosis through the use of healing properties of plants, such as herbs with anti-inflammatory effects. It is important to understand that while these herbs can help, they are not suitable for everyone and they can interfere with other medications and therapies.

Other approaches used in TCM include cupping, massages, moxibustion (burning herbal leaves near the body), and mind-body exercises like tai chi and yoga.

### Efficacy and Safety

TCM approaches may help patients who are looking for therapies that can help them better manage their symptoms during flare-ups. These therapies can also help reduce reliance on medications and boost overall musculoskeletal health.

Take acupuncture, for example. According to a 2023 review, this staple approach in Eastern medicine has shown strong benefits for spinal stenosis. (37) Not only does it play an important role in alleviating pain, improving quality of life, and decreasing disability, but it can also help patients who are facing the prospect of spinal surgery prepare for the intervention and benefit from shorter recovery times.

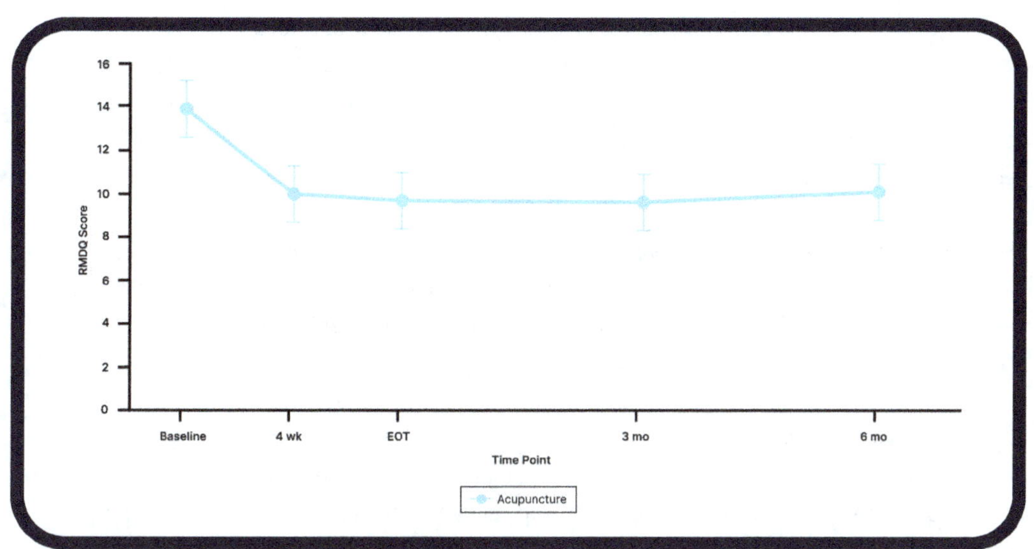


***Reduction of the Roland Morris Disability Questionnaire (RMDQ) score in patients with degenerative lumbar stenosis***
*Data from: https://www.amjmed.com/article/S0002-9343(19)30761-2/fulltext*

*The graph above shows the reduction of the Roland Morris Disability Questionnaire (RMDQ) score in patients with degenerative lumbar stenosis. The score is calculated at four weeks of treatment, at the end of treatment (EOT), and at three and six months after the treatment. The lower the RMDQ, the lower the disability perceived by the patient.*

Similarly, herbal remedies may be helpful in boosting blood circulation, reducing pain, and easing the swelling associated with inflammation. However, it is important to keep in mind that not all herbal remedies are adequately regulated and, just like nutraceuticals, they can interfere with the effects of important medications and lead to counterproductive effects on health. More studies are needed to determine the efficacy and safety of these approaches.

# Unconventional Surgical Procedures: Spinal Fusion

Spinal fusion is a surgical procedure that helps to correct issues affecting the vertebrae. It's essentially a "welding" process used to fuse together two or more vertebrae so they heal into a single, solid bone.

This process effectively eliminates the pain and inflammation associated with joint degeneration and movement. It can also be used to improve the stability of the spine or correct a deformity like the narrowing of the spinal canal. Your doctor might recommend spinal fusion if physical therapy, medications, or other non-invasive treatments haven't relieved your spinal stenosis.

New techniques - like minimally invasive spinal fusion surgery - have made this intervention a valid alternative to other more invasive options like laminectomy and laminotomy. Because of these developments, the number of spinal fusion surgeries performed on patients with spinal stenosis (with or without scoliosis) increased by nearly 15% between 2010 and 2014. (38)

### Efficacy and Safety

Fusion is a highly versatile intervention that can be used for a wide range of disorders. Since it eliminates the motion in the joints, it can help relieve pain and discomfort deriving from conditions like osteoarthritis and other inflammatory diseases. When used in the spine, this type of surgery shouldn't overly restrict movement and range of motion, but it can lead to some reduction in mobility.

This intervention also has some limitations. Firstly, studies have found that among patients with spinal stenosis, combining fusion surgery with standard decompression techniques (i.e. laminectomy and laminotomy) does not lead to better clinical outcomes than when decompression techniques are used alone. (39)

Additionally, spinal fusion is sometimes used to resolve the problem of spinal instability, which is a consequence of laminectomy or laminotomy. Nonetheless, the position of the World Federation of Neurosurgical Societies Spine Committee is that "fusion for instability or stenosis alone remains controversial, and the results are unconvincing." (40)

**Chapter 7 - Takeaways**

- Unconventional treatment options may be used in combination with other treatments to ease painful symptoms and reduce reliance on pain medications. Not all of them are equally effective or safe, and they should be administered only by specialists.
- Some of the nonsurgical unconventional treatment options that may help spinal stenosis include chiropractic and osteopathic care, nutraceuticals, diet and activity modification, and traditional Chinese medicine approaches (specifically herbal remedies and acupuncture).
- Other surgical options include spinal fusion, although some controversies still exist regarding the efficacy of this method.

# Chapter 8 - Stem Cell Treatment for Spinal Stenosis

Whether it's from a bone marrow aspirate concentration, adipose collection, or an expanded cell culture from perinatal tissue biologics, stem cell therapy is the most promising treatment for spinal stenosis that is already available in the US and around the world. The ultimate aspect that connects all these is that the concentration of cells needs to be high enough to produce an effective therapeutic outcome.

Currently, the only genuine high dose stem cell treatment for spinal stenosis in the US is via bone marrow aspirate concentrate, BMAC, or adipose collection. This is what I want to talk about first because it's here and now in the US medical market.

I want to say that if you're not eligible for a genuine high dose stem cell treatment using BMAC or adipose, there is always the high dose PRP option that is also a great treatment for spinal stenosis and other degenerative conditions of the spine, but this book is about stem cell treatments, and I'll review PRP options in detail in another book.

Bone marrow aspirate concentrate is the official standard source of genuine mesenchymal stem cells in the US medical market. This requires a fairly simple procedure where they aspirate bone marrow from a particular bone in your body, which may vary depending on the individual.

The doctor will likely decide which area is best for collection, and then process the bone marrow to isolate all the real mesenchymal stem cells and create a concentrated high dose injection of mesenchymal stem cells for injection into the damaged joint.

Remember earlier I discussed how the dose is everything? Well, it's still the case here later in the book: the dose is everything. One of the essential aspects of this process is measuring the quantity and viability of the cells collected and ensuring they are concentrated to an effective therapeutic level.

Much of this has been covered in earlier chapters – the different types of stem cells, how they work to treat conditions, and their increasing prevalence in medicine. Now that you have an increased understanding of stem cells, you might ask what evidence supports stem cell treatment for spinal stenosis. Relatively speaking, mesenchymal stem cell (MSC) treatment is straightforward.

For the most part, patients who undergo MSC treatment have noticeable pain relief through improved cartilage replacement, which ultimately leads to an enhanced quality of life. However, not all patients will elect to undergo MSC treatment without a deeper understanding of mesenchymal stem cell capability and function.

Mesenchymal stem cells have the capability to repair cartilage affected by osteoarthritis - thus reducing the risk of bulging discs and spinal stenosis - because they are able to target the affected areas, depending on the type of tissue in need of repair.

In the case of back pain caused by degenerative conditions of the spine, studies have found that even a single injection of bone marrow-derived mesenchymal stem cells (BMSCs) is safe and effective in reducing pain, limiting disability, and improving quality of life. (41)

Research published in 2021 also highlights the beneficial effects of stem cell therapy combined with an exercise program to address intervertebral disc degeneration and its complications (including spinal stenosis). (42)

## Cultured Expanded High Dose Stem Cells

As I explained previously, cultured expanded cell therapy refers to taking mesenchymal stem cells and growing them, or replicating them over and over to grow a much larger dose of cells.

You can't collect enough natural stem cells in an average bone marrow or adipose collection to treat multiple joints and conditions effectively, so the best way to get more cells is to grow them. The process is called cellular expansion. I've done cellular expansion work many times myself throughout my career in biotech and it's the true future of stem cell therapy.

You'll hear the term "expanded cell therapy," (or ECT) used to describe this process around the world by the medical and scientific community.

Unfortunately, expanded cell therapy is not permitted in the US and is only available out of the country. Despite it being the future of stem cell therapy, it's still difficult to regulate because there are many variables involved in the process.

Some of the most advanced research on expanded stem cells is occurring here in the US, but we can't offer the treatment to patients yet. I'm working actively to get this moving faster here in the US.

Earlier, I described two categories of stem cells: autologous and allogeneic. Autologous means your own cells, and allogeneic means a donor's cells. Some companies here in the US may collect bone marrow or adipose cells and offer to culture and expand them for treatment offered out of the country.

This has worked so far for many years, but the problem is that you need to have your cells collected, which is invasive in and of itself, and then you have to travel to get the treatment. If you're going to have to travel to get expanded cell therapy, you may as well avoid the invasive collection process and use qualified allogeneic stem cell sources that are younger cell lines.

Remember that if you're 70 years old and you collect your own stem cells, you're now using 70-year-old stem cells, and the growth capabilities and activity are limited. This doesn't mean those cells aren't useful, but it's obvious that new cell lines have an entire lifespan of activity ahead of them, so the overall understanding of this subject is that younger stem cells are better.

If you use allogeneic cell lines, you're using new age 0 stem cells with a full human life cycle of potential growth ahead of them. They are much more active and viable long-term, and this is why the future of stem cell therapy is using cultured expanded birth tissues.

As I explained earlier, we're talking about birth tissues from normal and ethical donation programs where the leftover tissues of regular C-section deliveries can be repurposed into medical therapies instead of being thrown in the medical trash bin.

This is from a healthy, regular pregnancy where the mother is screened and opts to donate these leftover tissues: the leftover amniotic fluid, placenta, cord tissue, cord blood, and amniotic membrane.

All of these materials would otherwise be disposed of after a C-section, but now we have a way to use them and advance medicine. I'd like to mention here that anyone who has donated tissues to this cause has advanced medical science and I applaud and respect your willingness to do this.

Leftover C-section tissue collection is perfectly harmless to the mother and newborn child, so it really is a matter of the mother being willing to allow this donation to happen, so again, I applaud and thank all the women who have volunteered to advance medical science! Thank you!

US regulations need to catch up with medical advancements so we can start doing advanced expanded cell therapy in the US. However, there are qualified medical centers around the world that are offering excellent expanded stem cell therapies.

Contact me directly and I'll refer you to the right places for this! Go to **willbozeman.com** and contact me there. Join my newsletter and other activities to learn all about what's going on in the world of stem cells.

DO NOT shop around for the cheapest options in questionable areas of the world. DO NOT use those medical tourism sites to shop, as they will readily let the worst treatment centers buy credibility on their platforms to get patients coming to them, or pay for promotion on those sites even though they are not the best locations for treatment.

There are literally no regulations on treatment centers in some areas. ALSO, I know for a fact that in some countries you can simply pay money to bypass regulations to get your medical certifications to set up a stem cell center. Or if you know someone or have a family member in government you can get permission to open a center without much oversight.

Be highly careful about where you go internationally for treatment.

I was launching a stem cell treatment center a few years ago, I can't say where for proprietary reasons, when one of the potential partners simply used family connections to bypass the regulations to set up the center. The requirement to do all this basically shifted control of the operation away from our US-based company and into the control of their local operation.

At that point, I just couldn't be involved because of the extreme risk of not being in control of the medical treatment process, so I exited the operation and have since worked with the top minds in the world on creating the most advanced and reputable stem cell treatment centers.

Some of these unscrupulous stem cell centers make wild claims and also, they can't document their cell sources and don't have all the right lab processing protocols, or at least they don't release that info to potential patients.

Again, if you want genuine expanded stem cell therapies, contact me and I'll direct you to the best centers around the world that are doing things the right way. There are excellent options, you just have to know where to go.

Because culture expanded stem cells are capable of expanding into other types of cells, this means they are also able to help various parts of the body like the heart or liver. More commonly, culture expanded mesenchymal stem cells are used in the regrowth of tissues and reduction of pain, but are they effective in treating spinal stenosis?

Firstly, this therapy has been seen to be effective in the treatment of osteoarthritis, which is a leading cause of spinal stenosis. Dr. Ricardo Bastos et al. conducted a study evaluating the efficacy and safety of culture expanded MSCs and platelet-rich plasma (PRP) when treating osteoarthritis.

These doctors and researchers were able to definitively conclude that, "[a]n intra-articular injection of bone marrow-derived culture-expanded MSCs with or without the [addition] of PRP is effective in improving the function and decreasing symptoms caused by knee OA at 12-month follow-up." (2020) (43)

Much like the implementation of BMAC stem cells, the level of efficacy patients experience correlates directly with the length of time they receive the treatment.

Additionally, a pilot study published in 2017 shows that the intradiscal injection of culture expanded MSCs to treat lumbar disc degeneration - which narrows the spinal canal - produced encouraging results, including no safety issues, substantially reduced pain, increased function, and reduced disc bulge size in most patients. (44)

The ultimate efficacy of these treatments also depended on the patient's adherence to doctor recommendations. For example, when a patient undergoes BMAC injections in the spine joints, mechanical support like braces may be recommended to reduce the stress load on the area treated and improve healing time.

These methods of treatment used in conjunction with the main procedure (being BMAC injection) might seem small, irritating, and unnecessary, but patients would do well to follow these recommendations to ensure the best possible outcomes.

In addition to treating spinal stenosis pain, patients can have a solid expectation that these stem cells will also address some of the root causes of spinal stenosis, like bulging discs, systemic inflammation, osteoarthritis, and OA-damaged cartilage.

As more and more patients with back pain find relief through stem cell treatment, there is more conclusive evidence to suggest that it is the next generation of pain treatment and musculoskeletal repair.

## Bank Your Own Stem Cells!

Even as an adult you can have your own stem cell cultured, expanded, and banked for future use. Using a simple adipose collection procedure, we can take a small sample of your fat tissue, isolate out the stem cells, and then grow them out in the lab to create dozens of vials of High Dose Stem Cells that are ideal for use down the road. Given the choice would you want to get a stem cell treatment with your own cells or a donor's cells? Most people would pick their own cells.

In the US it's not a standard treatment model yet to use your own cultured expanded stem cells, but you as a person can absolutely have your own cells grown and banked and own them yourself for the future. Once you own your own cells you can do what you want with them later on, so I like to point this out to people who are considering the future treatments that are coming around the corner in the US where it may be OK for people actively get stem cell treatments using their own cells that have been cultured, expanded and banked.

Reach out to me at willbozeman.com, or any of my social media accounts, and I'll connect you with labs that offer this service. Many of the top voices in the industry are already talking about the future acceptance of cultured expanded stem cell therapies in the US and it's going to be an asset for anyone who has their own cells ready to go!

# Chapter 9 - Recap and Solutions in the US and Solutions Internationally

Through my own research and review of the scientific data, throughout this book, I have shed light on the complex nature of degenerative spine conditions and their profound impact on those living with this potentially debilitating condition.

It's clear that spinal stenosis is a complex problem that presents a variety of challenges, such as chronic pain, limited movement, and diminishing quality of life for countless individuals all over the world.

Throughout the course of this book, you have learned a lot about the complexities of managing back pain and have become more educated about the promising alternatives that exist in the realm of stem cell therapies.

There is now a glimmer of hope for everyone looking for a way to alleviate the ongoing suffering and avoid the high-risk invasive surgical treatments associated with this condition, benefitting both individuals seeking relief as well as medical professionals searching for efficient treatments with longer-lasting results for patients under their care.

Through the chapters of this book, I have provided a thorough look at the current conventional treatment options available for spinal stenosis. This included the commonly prescribed NSAIDs and corticosteroid injections, as well as orthopedic surgical procedures.

While these approaches can offer varying degrees of relief, after this analysis, you are now aware of the limitations associated with these conventional treatments, including their underlying drawbacks and constraints. For instance, NSAIDs offer a temporary option that merely treats painful symptoms rather than addressing the underlying cause.

I have seen these often leave patients dependent on prolonged use of medications with the potential of developing negative side effects as a result. For some people, corticosteroid injections can provide moderate-term comfort; however, in my experience with variable success rates, limited duration of effectiveness, and high likelihood of repeat injections, they too have a number of disadvantages as well as a limited impact on health outcomes.

When seen as the last resort, surgical interventions represent a significant step for patients. It involves substantial recovery and rehabilitation periods as well as the notably heightened risks of complications. By the time this last resort surgical option becomes a possibility, patients have already undergone an exhausting and distressing process through the difficulties associated with spinal stenosis.

I have seen this currently implemented management journey leave patients in disheartening situations in which any hope for effective relief has faded, leaving them naturally hesitant to accept the dangers associated with surgical intervention. This important realization underscores to me the urgency for alternative approaches that offer relief without subjecting individuals to the risks and challenges of invasive procedures.

This exploration into stem cell therapies revealed that bone marrow aspirate concentrate (BMAC), adipose-derived stem cells, culture-expanded cells, and expanded cell therapy (ECT), all offer unique strengths with distinct advantages in healing and rejuvenating damaged tissues.

The essential takeaway from the findings of this regenerative therapy is that the concentration of stem cells is critical to achieving the greatest potential results and optimizing patient health outcomes.

There are some excellent options in the US market for all high dose stem cell therapy using BMAC and/or adipose stem cell therapy for regenerative medicine and spinal stenosis management.

Some groups that are standardizing their processes are offering the best options across the nation, with advanced techniques for stem cell therapies and other advanced regenerative therapies. Ultimately, stem cells and regenerative medicine are revolutionizing how spinal stenosis and its numerous challenges are managed.

To reiterate, conventional treatments for spinal stenosis only work for so long, and surgeries like laminectomy and laminotomy may create more problems than they solve. The ideal way to approach spinal stenosis and other degenerative conditions of the spine is with the least invasive options first.

Stem cells, platelet-rich plasma (PRP), platelet lysate (PL), and other injections are truly restructuring the way we treat spinal disorders, back pain, and other degenerative tissue conditions in the US and around the world.

I'd also like to point out that a good physician offering these treatments will likely offer musculoskeletal (MSK) ultrasound guidance and fluoroscopy techniques to guide their injections to the most targeted areas of damage.

Traditional medical providers who have a lot of experience don't necessarily need image guidance for injection into large joints, but many of them will acknowledge they prefer to use guidance for surety because it's good medical practice. Relying on landmarks and going with "blind" injections isn't ideal, especially if you're paying a lot for the treatment.

You want the best possible outcome, so use the best techniques to obtain it and minimize the element of guesswork. MSK ultrasound provides real-time images of the joint, while fluoroscopy also provides X-ray video that offers a clearer and more comprehensive view. Together, these technologies are excellent and you should look for offices that utilize these image guidance measures.

Where to go in the US for the right treatments?

Visit my website at willbozeman.com or contact me through any of my social media platforms and I'll send you to the best possible location nearest to you where you can get the best options. I know you may be tempted to just search the internet for this, but I know for a fact that some of the worst players in the field of regenerative medicine have some of the best marketing!

So, doing a search in your area will likely bring up several great options, but only a few of them may actually be great and the rest may be either average or inferior, even if the cost is lower. REMEMBER, it's the quality of the injection as well as the delivery of the injection that make it work! Just because an office is promoting an inexpensive stem cell or PRP injection doesn't mean it's a good option.

If the concentration isn't high enough you won't trigger the regenerative effect and suddenly even that lower priced treatment is WAY overpriced for the benefit you gained. It's much better to pay the extra for a good provider and get the real deal, high dose stem cells and high dose PRP!

Can you imagine a future where OA pain doesn't define your day? Or a future where every movement isn't considered for how much pain it will cause? Also, a future where surgery and joint replacements are no longer the default solution, but a rare occurrence for the worst cases?

Where to go for international stem cell treatment centers?

Connect with me on willbozeman.com or my social media accounts and reach out to me directly and I'll get you to the right locations and the best centers with the most reliable providers and therapies.

I don't want to mention any particular center or group here because the international market is always changing and the providers in those centers also change, and an endorsement in writing can last long after that center loses its status and acceptance as a top level International Stem Cell Treatment Center.

Obviously, I've already spent time reviewing all this with you but I want to recap this again. The best option for genuine stem cell therapy and the future of stem cell therapy is using cultured expanded stem cells from perinatal birth tissues.

It's the most promising option for wide-scale application and convenience. Also, I'm confident that in the coming years this treatment will be refined and standardized and entered into the US market. Also, with scale comes cost and price reduction, allowing for further scale and wider participation. I'm very excited about this.

Until then, be highly careful about where you go and how you are referred there. Online searches are sometimes dangerous and international medical tourism sites can be bought and paid for by the bad actors.

I'm happy to connect you with the best option for the treatment you need by connecting with me on my website willbozeman.com and simply asking me where you should go for treatment. Let's all work together to make stem cell therapy the future of medicine!

# Conclusion

By now you have learned quite a bit more than most people know or understand about stem cells and stem cell therapy options inside and outside the US medical market.

Also, I hope you know more about some of the other excellent non-stem cell options available here in the US that are still excellent starting points for anyone suffering from a degenerative spine condition. Remember that a really good PRP is an excellent option as well and that is available here in the US and I can direct you to the right location for that.

Your options in the US are tremendous, so I don't want anyone to think that they can't get some of the best treatments in the world here in the US. The expanded cell therapy market outside the US is much more expensive and difficult to navigate, so I don't like telling people to just go get the latest and greatest from anywhere in the world.

I want to make sure those options are vetted, so people asking me are going to the right places. Always reach out to me on my personal site to ask about where to go for whatever you're looking for.

My experience in the biotech field and in owning and operating multiple biotech labs and medical practices and various other lab companies has helped me appreciate the complexity of this new era of stem cell therapy. I'm confident in the future of medicine and what we can accomplish.

It may be scary to some, but after years of seeing doctors and patients warm up to the new therapy options, and seeing the results, I'm confident that a new wave of acceptance in stem cell therapy will continue to trigger new advancements in the field.

I maintain connections across the nation and the world on regenerative medicine to keep my finger on the pulse of what's going on and what is being developed.

If you are uncertain about what you're being told, or what you're reading, the promises of cure and treatment being presented, or even the price of the therapy being offered, reach out to me and I'll help guide you. I can dig into just about any marketing pitch from any practice and see what they are actually offering.

I may not be able to advocate for you directly, but I can help guide you on your journey. At the very least I can send you to people who I know will take care of you properly and not simply recite some marketing material to you or promise you the world and a lifetime of health and happiness for a swipe of your credit card. Let's work together to make regenerative medicine the field it's meant to be and advocate for the good and eliminate the bad. We can do it together!

I look forward to seeing, talking, and connecting with you directly on my personal site willbozeman.com, as well as any of my social media accounts:

- Twitter: @WBozeman70246
- Facebook: @WillBozemanCEO
- LinkedIn: @will-bozeman
- Instagram: @willbozemanceo

Thank you so much for reading this book and taking the leap to learn more about this new era of medicine. My last request is that after you have read this book and you've connected with me to guide you on where to go for treatment, give this book to someone else who's suffering from spinal stenosis. Every little thing we can do for one of us will help all of us!

# References


1. Hsiang, J. K. (n.d.). Spinal Stenosis: Practice Essentials, Anatomy, Pathophysiology. https://emedicine.medscape.com/article/1913265-overview#

2. Krebs EE, Lurie JD, Fanciullo G, Tosteson TD, Blood EA, Carey TS, Weinstein JN. Predictors of long-term opioid use among patients with painful lumbar spine conditions. J Pain. 2010 Jan;11(1):44-52. doi: 10.1016/j.jpain.2009.05.007. Epub 2009 Jul 22. PMID: 19628436; PMCID: PMC2818028.

3. Kim JE, Choi DJ, Park EJJ, Lee HJ, Hwang JH, Kim MC, Oh JS. Biportal Endoscopic Spinal Surgery for Lumbar Spinal Stenosis. Asian Spine J. 2019 Apr;13(2):334-342. doi: 10.31616/asj.2018.0210. Epub 2019 Apr 30. PMID: 30959588; PMCID: PMC6454273.

4. Deer T, Sayed D, Michels J, Josephson Y, Li S, Calodney AK. A Review of Lumbar Spinal Stenosis with Intermittent Neurogenic Claudication: Disease and Diagnosis. Pain Med. 2019 Dec 1;20(Suppl 2):S32-S44. doi: 10.1093/pm/pnz161. PMID: 31808530; PMCID: PMC7101166.

5. 1.00 Musculoskeletal Disorders - Adult. (n.d.). https://www.ssa.gov/disability/professionals/bluebook/1.00-Musculoskeletal-Adult.htm

6. Parenteau CS, Lau EC, Campbell IC, Courtney A. Prevalence of spine degeneration diagnosis by type, age, gender, and obesity using Medicare data. Sci Rep. 2021 Mar 8;11(1):5389. doi: 10.1038/s41598-021-84724-6. PMID: 33686128; PMCID: PMC7940625.

7. Kalff R, Ewald C, Waschke A, Gobisch L, Hopf C. Degenerative lumbar spinal stenosis in older people: current treatment options. Dtsch Arztebl Int. 2013 Sep;110(37):613-23; quiz 624. doi: 10.3238/arztebl.2013.0613. Epub 2013 Sep 13. PMID: 24078855; PMCID: PMC3784039.

8. Chen Z, Luo R, Yang Y, Xiang Z. The prevalence of depression in degenerative spine disease patients: A systematic review and meta-analysis. Eur Spine J. 2021 Dec;30(12):3417-3427. doi: 10.1007/s00586-021-06977-z. Epub 2021 Sep 2. PMID: 34476597.


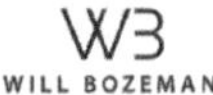

9. Surgery for spinal stenosis linked to lower mortality and costs. (2023, January 13). https://www.wolterskluwer.com/en/news/surgery-for-spinal-stenosis-linked-to-lower-mortality-and-costs

10. Munakomi, S. (2023, August 13). Spinal Stenosis and Neurogenic Claudication. StatPearls - NCBI Bookshelf. https://www.ncbi.nlm.nih.gov/books/NBK430872/

11. Battié, M. C., Jones, C. A., Schopflocher, D. P., & Hu, R. W. (2012, March). Health-related quality of life and comorbidities associated with lumbar spinal stenosis. The Spine Journal, 12(3), 189–195. https://doi.org/10.1016/j.spinee.2011.11.009

12. Koes BW, van Tulder MW, Peul WC. Diagnosis and treatment of sciatica. BMJ. 2007 Jun 23;334(7607):1313-7. doi: 10.1136/bmj.39223.428495.BE. PMID: 17585160; PMCID: PMC1895638.

13. Kalichman L, Cole R, Kim DH, Li L, Suri P, Guermazi A, Hunter DJ. Spinal stenosis prevalence and association with symptoms: the Framingham Study. Spine J. 2009 Jul;9(7):545-50. doi: 10.1016/j.spinee.2009.03.005. Epub 2009 Apr 23. PMID: 19398386; PMCID: PMC3775665.

14. Inflammation: A unifying theory of disease? (2023, March 29). Harvard Health. https://www.health.harvard.edu/staying-healthy/inflammation-a-unifying-theory-of-disease

15. Raja, A. (2023, June 12). Spinal Stenosis. StatPearls - NCBI Bookshelf. https://www.ncbi.nlm.nih.gov/books/NBK441989/

16. Rajesh N, Moudgil-Joshi J, Kaliaperumal C. Smoking and degenerative spinal disease: A systematic review. Brain Spine. 2022 Aug 7;2:100916. doi: 10.1016/j.bas.2022.100916. PMID: 36248118; PMCID: PMC9560562.

17. Casiano, V. E. (2023, February 20). Back Pain. StatPearls - NCBI Bookshelf. https://www.ncbi.nlm.nih.gov/books/NBK538173/

18. Yang H, Hurwitz EL, Li J, de Luca K, Tavares P, Green B, Haldeman S. Bidirectional Comorbid Associations between Back Pain and Major Depression in US Adults. Int J Environ Res Public Health. 2023 Feb 27;20(5):4217. doi: 10.3390/ijerph20054217. PMID: 36901226; PMCID: PMC10002070.

19. Wu, Y., Zhang, Z., Wang, F. et al. Current status of traumatic spinal cord injury caused by traffic accident in Northern China. Sci Rep 12, 13892 (2022). https://doi.org/10.1038/s41598-022-16930-9

20. Elmasry S, Asfour S, de Rivero Vaccari JP, Travascio F. Effects of Tobacco Smoking on the Degeneration of the Intervertebral Disc: A Finite Element Study. PLoS One. 2015 Aug 24;10(8):e0136137. doi: 10.1371/journal.pone.0136137. PMID: 26301590; PMCID: PMC4547737.

21. Luoma K, Riihimäki H, Raininko R, Luukkonen R, Lamminen A, Viikari-Juntura E. Lumbar disc degeneration in relation to occupation. Scand J Work Environ Health. 1998 Oct;24(5):358-66. doi: 10.5271/sjweh.356. PMID: 9869307.

22. Pollard, H., Hansen, L. & Hoskins, W. Cervical stenosis in a professional rugby league football player: a case report . Chiropr Man Therap 13, 15 (2005). https://doi.org/10.1186/1746-1340-13-15

23. Hwang, R. W., Briggs, C. M., Greenwald, S. D., Manberg, P. J., Chamoun, N. G., & Tromanhauser, S. G. (2023, January 12). Surgical Treatment of Single-Level Lumbar Stenosis Is Associated with Lower 2-Year Mortality and Total Cost Compared with Nonsurgical Treatment. Journal of Bone and Joint Surgery, 105(3), 214–222. https://doi.org/10.2106/jbjs.22.00181

24. Duncan JW, Bailey RA. Cauda equina syndrome following decompression for spinal stenosis. Global Spine J. 2011 Dec;1(1):15-8. doi: 10.1055/s-0031-1296051. PMID: 24353932; PMCID: PMC3864468.

25. Marcum ZA, Hanlon JT. Recognizing the Risks of Chronic Nonsteroidal Anti-Inflammatory Drug Use in Older Adults. Ann Longterm Care. 2010;18(9):24-27. PMID: 21857795; PMCID: PMC3158445.

26. Leonie H. A. Broersen, Alberto M. Pereira, Jens Otto L. Jørgensen, Olaf M. Dekkers, Adrenal Insufficiency in Corticosteroids Use: Systematic Review and Meta-Analysis, The Journal of Clinical Endocrinology & Metabolism, Volume 100, Issue 6, 1 June 2015, Pages 2171–2180, https://doi.org/10.1210/jc.2015-1218

27. Chen X, Gan Y, Li W, Su J, Zhang Y, Huang Y, Roberts AI, Han Y, Li J, Wang Y, Shi Y. The interaction between mesenchymal stem cells and steroids during inflammation. Cell Death Dis. 2014 Jan 23;5(1):e1009. doi: 10.1038/cddis.2013.537. PMID: 24457953; PMCID: PMC4040685.

28. Sullivan, M. D., & Ballantyne, J. C. (2023, July). Randomised trial reveals opioids relieve acute back pain no better than placebo. The Lancet, 402(10398), 267–269. https://doi.org/10.1016/s0140-6736(23)00671-2

29. Nunley PD, Deer TR, Benyamin RM, Staats PS, Block JE. Interspinous process decompression is associated with a reduction in opioid analgesia in patients with lumbar spinal stenosis. J Pain Res. 2018 Nov 20;11:2943-2948. doi: 10.2147/JPR.S182322. PMID: 30538533; PMCID: PMC6251434.

30. Bartels RH, Groenewoud H, Peul WC, Arts MP. Lamifuse: results of a randomized controlled trial comparing laminectomy with and without fusion for cervical spondylotic myelopathy. J Neurosurg Sci. 2017 Apr;61(2):134-139. doi: 10.23736/S0390-5616.16.03315-4. Epub 2015 Jun 17. PMID: 26082384.

31. Bydon M, Macki M, De la Garza-Ramos R, McGovern K, Sciubba DM, Wolinsky JP, Witham TF, Gokaslan ZL, Bydon A. Incidence of Adjacent Segment Disease Requiring Reoperation After Lumbar Laminectomy Without Fusion: A Study of 398 Patients. Neurosurgery. 2016 Feb;78(2):192-9. doi: 10.1227/NEU.0000000000001007. PMID: 26348008.

32. Haddadi K, Ganjeh Qazvini HR. Outcome after Surgery of Lumbar Spinal Stenosis: A Randomized Comparison of Bilateral Laminotomy, Trumpet Laminectomy, and Conventional Laminectomy. Front Surg. 2016 Apr 8;3:19. doi: 10.3389/fsurg.2016.00019. PMID: 27092304; PMCID: PMC4824790.

33. Kim TH, Lee BH, Lee HM, Lee SH, Park JO, Kim HS, Kim SW, Moon SH. Prevalence of vitamin D deficiency in patients with lumbar spinal stenosis and its relationship with pain. Pain Physician. 2013 Mar-Apr;16(2):165-76. PMID: 23511683.

34. Glucosamine and Chondroitin for Osteoarthritis. (n.d.). NCCIH. https://www.nccih.nih.gov/health/glucosamine-and-chondroitin-for-osteoarthritis-what-you-need-to-know#

35. Turner RC, Lucke-Wold BP, Boo S, Rosen CL, Sedney CL. The potential dangers of neck manipulation & risk for dissection and devastating stroke: An illustrative case & review of the literature. Biomed Res Rev. 2018;2(1):10.15761/BRR.1000110. doi: 10.15761/BRR.1000110. Epub 2018 Mar 25. PMID: 29951644; PMCID: PMC6016850.

36. Verhaeghe N, Schepers J, van Dun P, Annemans L. Osteopathic care for spinal complaints: A systematic literature review. PLoS One. 2018 Nov 2;13(11):e0206284. doi: 10.1371/journal.pone.0206284. Erratum in: PLoS One. 2019 Aug 8;14(8):e0221140. PMID: 30388155; PMCID: PMC6214527.

37. Clark A, Lucke-Wold BP. Acupuncture and Spinal Stenosis: Considerations for Treatment. Futur Integr Med. 2022 Dec;1(1):23-31. doi: 10.14218/fim.2022.00010. Epub 2022 May 31. PMID: 36705625; PMCID: PMC9875941.

38. Reisener MJ, Pumberger M, Shue J, Girardi FP, Hughes AP. Trends in lumbar spinal fusion-a literature review. J Spine Surg. 2020 Dec;6(4):752-761. doi: 10.21037/jss-20-492. PMID: 33447679; PMCID: PMC7797794.

39. Försth, P., Ólafsson, G., Carlsson, T., Frost, A., Borgström, F., Fritzell, P., Öhagen, P., Michaëlsson, K., & Sandén, B. (2016, April 14). A Randomized, Controlled Trial of Fusion Surgery for Lumbar Spinal Stenosis. New England Journal of Medicine, 374(15), 1413–1423. https://doi.org/10.1056/nejmoa1513721

40. Sharif S, Shaikh Y, Bajamal AH, Costa F, Zileli M. Fusion Surgery for Lumbar Spinal Stenosis: WFNS Spine Committee Recommendations. World Neurosurg X. 2020 Mar 18;7:100077. doi: 10.1016/j.wnsx.2020.100077. PMID: 32613190; PMCID: PMC7322802.

41. Sudo H, Miyakoshi T, Watanabe Y, Ito YM, Kahata K, Tha KK, Yokota N, Kato H, Terada T, Iwasaki N, Arato T, Sato N, Isoe T. Protocol for treating lumbar spinal canal stenosis with a combination of ultrapurified, allogenic bone marrow-derived mesenchymal stem cells and in situ-forming gel: a multicentre, prospective, double-blind randomised controlled trial. BMJ Open. 2023 Feb 2;13(2):e065476. doi: 10.1136/bmjopen-2022-065476. PMID: 36731929; PMCID: PMC9896178.

42. Li B, Yang Y, Wang L, Liu G. Stem Cell Therapy and Exercise for Treatment of Intervertebral Disc Degeneration. Stem Cells Int. 2021 Oct 13;2021:7982333. doi: 10.1155/2021/7982333. PMID: 34691192; PMCID: PMC8528633.

43. Bastos R, Mathias M, Andrade R, Amaral RJFC, Schott V, Balduino A, Bastos R, Miguel Oliveira J, Reis RL, Rodeo S, Espregueira-Mendes J. Intra-articular injection of culture-expanded mesenchymal stem cells with or without addition of platelet-rich plasma is effective in decreasing pain and symptoms in knee osteoarthritis: a controlled, double-blind clinical trial. Knee Surg Sports Traumatol Arthrosc. 2020 Jun;28(6):1989-1999. doi: 10.1007/s00167-019-05732-8. Epub 2019 Oct 5. PMID: 31587091.

44. Centeno C, Markle J, Dodson E, Stemper I, Williams CJ, Hyzy M, Ichim T, Freeman M. Treatment of lumbar degenerative disc disease-associated radicular pain with culture-expanded autologous mesenchymal stem cells: a pilot study on safety and efficacy. J Transl Med. 2017 Sep 22;15(1):197. doi: 10.1186/s12967-017-1300-y. PMID: 28938891; PMCID: PMC5610473.

www.ingramcontent.com/pod-product-compliance
Lightning Source LLC
LaVergne TN
LVHW010613110826
845149LV00003B/885

* 9 7 8 1 9 6 3 5 9 2 1 0 8 *